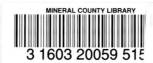

Mayo Clinic on Chronic Pain provides reliable, practical information on managing chronic pain. Much of the information comes directly from the experience of pain specialists and other health care professionals at Mayo Clinic. This book supplements the advice of your physician, whom you should consult for individual medical problems. *Mayo Clinic on Chronic Pain* does not endorse any company or product. MAYO, MAYO CLINIC, MAYO CLINIC HEALTH INFORMATION and the Mayo triple-shield logo are marks of Mayo Foundation for Medical Education and Research.

Published by Mayo Clinic Health Information, Rochester, Minn. Distributed to the book trade by Kensington Publishing Corporation, New York, N.Y.

Photo credits: Cover photos and the photos on pages 1, 45 and 99 are from PhotoDisc®.

Library of Congress Catalog Card Number 2002104998

ISBN 1-893005-27-5

Printed in the United States of America

Second Edition

4 5 6 7 8 9 10

About chronic pain

Chronic pain is a major cause of distress, despair and disability in the United States and around the world. It affects men, women and children in all walks of life. Chronic pain may involve a specific region of your body, such as your head or lower back, or it can affect your entire body, as it does with the generalized pain disorder called fibromyalgia.

Chronic pain is by its very nature a long-term health problem for most people who have it. Many treatments are available, some of which are well researched, safe and effective. Other available treatments have not been thoroughly tested, may not be widely accepted or may have significant risks and side effects.

Scientific research taking place in medical centers and laboratories around the world holds much promise for future advances in the understanding and treatment of chronic pain. But most important, information, treatments and rehabilitative therapies that are available today can help you to feel better, to improve your quality of life and to return to more normal function if you struggle with chronic pain.

About Mayo Clinic

Mayo Clinic evolved from the frontier practice of Dr. William Worrall Mayo and the partnership of his two sons, William J. and Charles H. Mayo, in the early 1900s. Pressed by the demands of their busy practice in Rochester, Minn., the Mayo brothers invited other physicians to join them, pioneering the private group practice of medicine. Today, with more than 2,000 physicians and scientists at its three major locations in Rochester, Minn., Jacksonville, Fla., and Scottsdale, Ariz., Mayo Clinic is dedicated to providing comprehensive diagnoses, accurate answers and effective treatments.

With this depth of medical knowledge, experience and expertise, Mayo Clinic occupies an unparalleled position as a health information resource. Since 1983 Mayo Clinic has published reliable health information for millions of consumers through a variety of award-winning newsletters, books and online services. Revenue from these publishing activities supports Mayo Clinic programs, including medical education and medical research.

Editorial staff

Editor in Chief
Jeffrey Rome, M.D.

Contributing Medical Editors
John E. Hodgson, L.P.
Connie Luedtke, R.N.

Managing Editor
Richard Dietman

Editorial Research
Anthony Cook
Deirdre Herman
Michelle Hewlett

Proofreading
Miranda Attlesey
Louise Filipic
Donna Hanson

Contributing Writers
Anne Christiansen
Rebecca Gonzalez-Campoy
D.R. Martin
Stephen Miller
Doug Toft
Susan Wichmann

Creative Director
Daniel Brevick

Layout and Production
Craig King

Illustration and Photography
John Hagen
Michael King
Kent McDaniel
Christopher Srnka
Rebecca Varga

Indexing
Larry Harrison

Contributing editors and reviewers

Julie Abbott, M.D.
John Bartleson, M.D.
Susan Bee, R.N., C.N.S.
Tracy Berg, R.Ph.
Ines Berger, M.D.
Adil Bharucha, M.D.
Barbara Bruce, Ph.D.
Mark Canny, O.T.R.
Kaye Ebnet, R.N.
Stephen Erickson, M.D.
Michele Evans, R.N., C.N.S.
Christopher Frye
Thomas Gauvin
Andrew Good, M.D.
Heather Hansen, O.T.R.
Connie Hollister, R.N.
Marc Huntoon, M.D.
Susan Klingsporn, R.N.
David Martin, M.D.
Jennifer K. Nelson, R.D.
Pamela Nelson, R.N., C.N.S.

Laura Newell, R.N.
Jennifer O'Conner, C.O.T.A.
Karen Olson, R.D.
John Postier, P.T.
Kevin Reid, D.M.D.
Karla Resch, O.T.R.
Andrea Reynolds, R.P.T.
Lizabeth Roers, C.O.T.A.
Howard Rome, Ph.D.
Scott Ross, D.O.
Paola Sandroni, M.D.
Christopher Sletten, Ph.D.
Lisa Solie, O.T.R.
Jeffrey M. Thompson, M.D.
Wendy N. Timm, P.T.
Tamra Trenary, O.T.R.
Lori Turba Rogers, O.T.R.
Susan Utesch, R.N.
Merri Vitse, C.O.T.A.
Mikel Wheeler, O.T.R.

Preface

Accurate and useful information is vital to maintaining good health and managing illness. This is particularly true for the common and often-complicated problem of chronic pain. The first edition of *Mayo Clinic on Chronic Pain* was published in 1999 to provide reliable information on this subject. The first edition has been a very popular part of Mayo Clinic's collection of health-related publications and has been translated into six languages.

Advances in the field of pain medicine are occurring rapidly and are the driving force behind publication of this second edition. This updated book, like the first edition, provides information on how the nervous system responds to painful illnesses and injuries and describes common painful conditions such as migraines, low back pain and fibromyalgia. This second edition has expanded sections on medications used for pain and on interventional treatments such as spinal cord stimulators and pain pumps.

This book emphasizes a take-charge approach to successfully managing chronic pain by providing detailed information and instructions on exercise, daily activities and stress reduction techniques. Complementary and alternative medicine approaches for coping with chronic pain also are reviewed, and there's new information on the process of nervous system sensitization to pain signals.

The expertise of Mayo Clinic physicians, psychologists, nurses, and physical and occupational therapists is the foundation of the pain management strategies presented in this book. I'm indebted to the staff of Mayo Clinic's Pain Rehabilitation Center, Pain Clinic and Fibromyalgia Treatment Program for their assistance in producing this second edition of *Mayo Clinic on Chronic Pain.*

We believe you'll find this book to be a practical resource for effectively managing chronic pain. Your knowledge and use of pain management strategies, together with the support of family and friends and the guidance of your personal physician, offer you the best opportunity to overcome the problem of chronic pain.

Jeffrey Rome, M.D.
Editor in Chief

Contents

Part 1: Understanding chronic pain

Part 2: Treating chronic pain

Part 3: Managing chronic pain

Part 1

Understanding chronic pain

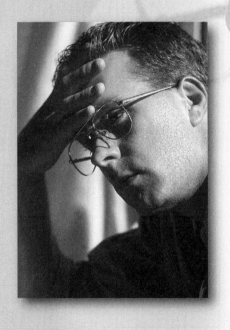

Chapter 1

What is pain?

Pain is a universal experience. We all feel it, whether it's the sharp, stabbing pain of a twisted ankle or the deep, throbbing pain of a headache that won't quit. Pain knows no age limit — it affects us from infancy through old age. Almost half of all Americans seek treatment for pain each year, 7 million from newly diagnosed back pain alone.

Sensitivity to pain is complex and varies from person to person. An experience that for one person causes immediate, excruciating pain may for another result in only minor discomfort. And this varied sensitivity can sometimes make pain hard to describe. The degree to which you feel pain and how you react to it are the results of your biological, psychological and cultural makeup. And your past encounters with painful injury or illness also can have an influence on your sensitivity to pain.

There are times when pain can be useful — almost protective — such as when it warns you that the hot skillet you've just picked up will burn your hand if you don't put it down quickly. But other pain — the day-after-day chronic ache of arthritis or the constant throbbing of a headache — seems to serve no useful purpose. And its relentlessness can be overwhelming.

When pain persists beyond the time expected for an injury to heal or an illness to end, it can become a chronic condition.

No longer is the pain viewed as just the symptom of another disease, but as an illness unto itself. This type of pain is commonly referred to as chronic pain or chronic noncancer pain in order to distinguish it from cancer (malignant) pain. It may also be called chronic benign pain, though nothing about it may seem benign.

Unfortunately, chronic pain can be difficult to treat. Strategies on how best to manage it are the subject of much research currently under way at medical centers around the world. In most instances, a comprehensive approach that may include medication, nerve stimulation, exercise, relaxation training and behavioral change is used in treating chronic pain. Medication alone is usually not sufficient to help people who struggle to cope with chronic pain. The good news is that despite having persistent pain, you can still have an active, productive and satisfying lifestyle.

Managing chronic pain has evolved from a time when it was thought that pain was something to be tolerated and endured, and that complaining or seeking relief was a sign of weakness. But medical practice has determined that pain is something that must be considered when evaluating the basic condition of a person seeking medical care. Indeed, pain has been termed the fifth vital sign by the American Pain Society, and doctors are urged to assess their patients for pain every time they check them for pulse, blood pressure, body temperature and respiration.

The U.S. Congress has declared the current decade the Decade of Pain Control and Research. And the Joint Commission on Accreditation of Healthcare Organizations (JCAHO), which sets and

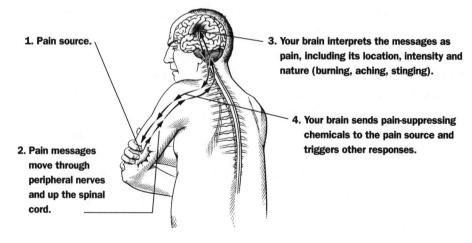

1. Pain source.

2. Pain messages move through peripheral nerves and up the spinal cord.

3. Your brain interprets the messages as pain, including its location, intensity and nature (burning, aching, stinging).

4. Your brain sends pain-suppressing chemicals to the pain source and triggers other responses.

Making sense of your nervous system

Your nervous system is composed of nerve cells and fibers that transmit and receive messages in the form of electrical currents and chemical interactions. It's through this intricate web of cells that your body and brain communicate.

Two main components make up your nervous system: your central nervous system, which includes your brain and spinal cord, and your peripheral nervous system. Your peripheral nerves extend from your spinal cord to your skin, muscles and internal organs. Within each of these systems are three major categories of nerves:

- Autonomic nerves maintain normal body processes, such as breathing, heart rate, blood pressure, digestion, perspiration and sexual function.
- Motor nerves are responsible for movement of your muscles. They allow you to move your hands and feet, to walk or sit.
- Sensory nerves are your sensing nerves. They allow you to feel an object when you touch it. They're also the nerves that allow you to feel pain.

enforces standards of care in hospitals and other health care facilities, has a list of 10 standards designed to ensure that the assessment and treatment of pain are part of the care of every patient.

This book can help you better understand your pain and its harmful effects, and perhaps more importantly, it explains how you can take control of your pain — instead of letting it control you.

How you feel pain

Understanding how your body feels pain can help you appreciate how you experience pain. It can also help you better understand why chronic pain is often difficult to treat.

Pain basically results from a series of electrical and chemical exchanges involving three major components: your peripheral nerves, spinal cord and brain.

Your peripheral nerves

Your peripheral (pe-RIF-er-ul) nerves encompass a network of nerve fibers that branches throughout your body. Attached to some of these fibers are special nerve endings that can sense an unpleasant stimulus, such as a cut, burn or painful pressure. These nerve endings are called nociceptors (no-sih-SEP-turs).

You have millions of nociceptors in your skin, bones, joints and muscles and in the protective membrane around your internal organs. Nociceptors are concentrated in areas more prone to injury, such as your fingers and toes. That's why a splinter in your finger hurts more than one in your back or shoulder. There may be as many as 1,300 nociceptors in just 1 square inch of skin. Muscles, protected beneath your skin, have fewer nerve endings. And internal organs, protected by skin, muscle and bone, have fewer still.

Some nociceptors sense sharp blows, others heat. One type senses pressure, temperature and chemical changes. Nociceptors can also detect inflammation caused by injury, disease or infection.

When nociceptors detect a harmful stimulus, they relay their pain messages in the form of electrical impulses along a peripheral nerve to your spinal cord and brain. However, the speed by which the messages travel can vary. Sensations of severe pain are transmitted almost instantaneously. Dull, aching pain — such as an upset stomach or an earache — is relayed on fibers that transmit at a slower speed.

Your spinal cord

When pain messages reach your spinal cord, they meet up with specialized nerve cells that act as gatekeepers, which filter the pain messages on their way to your brain.

For severe pain that's linked to bodily harm, such as when you touch a hot stove, the "gate" is wide open and the messages take an express route to your brain. Nerve cells in your spinal cord also respond to these urgent warnings by triggering other parts of the nervous system into action, such as your motor nerves. Your motor nerves signal your muscles to pull your hand away from the burner. Weak pain messages, however, such as from a scratch, may be filtered or blocked out by the gate.

Within your spinal cord, the messages can also change. Other sensations may overpower and diminish the pain signals. This happens when you massage or apply pressure to the injured area. The result is that the warnings sent by your peripheral nerves are downgraded to a lower priority.

Nerve cells in your spinal cord may also release chemicals that amplify or diminish the messages, affecting the strength of the pain signal that reaches your brain.

Your brain

When pain messages reach your brain, they arrive at the thalamus, a sorting and switching station located deep inside your brain. The thalamus quickly interprets the messages as pain and forwards them simultaneously to three specialized regions of the brain: the physical sensation region (somatosensory cortex), the emotional feeling region (limbic system) and the thinking region (frontal cortex). Your awareness of pain is therefore a complex experience of sensing, feeling and thinking.

Your brain responds to pain by sending messages that promote the healing process. For instance, if you've cut your finger, it signals your autonomic nervous system, the system that controls blood flow, to send additional blood and nutrients to the injury site. It also dispatches the release of pain-suppressing chemicals and sends stop-pain messages to the injury site.

Your pain response

When pain messages reach your brain, two components determine how you respond.

Physical sensation

Pain comes in many forms: sharp, jabbing, throbbing, burning, stinging, tingling, nagging, dull and aching. Pain also varies from mild to severe. Severe pain grabs your attention more quickly and generally produces a greater physical and emotional response than mild pain. Severe pain can also incapacitate you, making it difficult or impossible to sit or stand.

Natural painkillers and pain enhancers

Your brain and spinal cord produce their own painkillers, which are similar to the narcotic drug morphine, used to treat severe pain. Two of these morphine-like pain relievers are called endorphins (en-DOR-fins) and enkephalins (en-KEF-uh-lins). When released, these substances attach to special receptors in your brain, producing stop-pain messages.

Other substances in your body do just the opposite. They intensify your pain. A protein called substance P stimulates nerve endings at the injury site and within your spinal cord, increasing pain messages. Other pain enhancers work by activating normally silent nerve cells in the injured area. The activation of the silent nerve cells prompts the cells to discharge pain messages even when the stimulation they detect isn't painful. This not only worsens the pain but also enlarges the area of sensitivity.

The location of your pain also can affect your response to it. A headache that interferes with your ability to work or concentrate may be more bothersome — and therefore receive a stronger response — than arthritic pain in your knee or a cut to your finger.

Personal makeup

Your emotional and psychological state, memories of past pain experiences, and your upbringing and attitude also affect how you interpret pain messages and tolerate pain.

For example, a minor sensation that would barely register as pain, such as a dentist's probe, can actually produce exaggerated pain for a child who's never been to the dentist and who's heard horror stories about what it's like.

But your emotional state can also work in your favor, improving even a severe pain experience. This was illustrated by a study that compared formerly wounded war veterans with men in the general population. Men in both groups had the same kind of surgery. The combat veterans, however, required less pain medication than the others did, perhaps because they thought that the surgery was a minor matter compared with what they'd experienced in battle.

Athletes also can condition themselves to endure pain that would incapacitate others. In addition, if you were raised in a home or culture that taught you to "Grin and bear it" or to "Bite the bullet," you may experience less discomfort than people who focus on their pain or who are more prone to complain.

Acute pain and chronic pain

Acute pain is triggered by tissue damage. It's the type of pain that generally accompanies illness, injury or surgery.

Acute pain may be mild and last just a moment, such as from a sting. Or it can be severe and last for weeks or months, such as from a burn, pulled muscle or broken bone.

When you have acute pain, you know exactly where it hurts. In fact, the word *acute* comes from the Latin word for "needle," referring to a sharp pain. A toothache from a cavity, a burning elbow from a scrape and pain from a surgical incision are examples of acute pain. In a fairly predictable period and with treatment of the underlying cause, acute pain generally fades away — when the cavity is filled, the skin grows back or the incision heals.

Chronic pain hangs on after the injury is healed. Pain is generally described as chronic when it lasts 6 months or longer. This is reflected in the word itself. *Chronic* comes from the Greek word for "time."

As with acute pain, chronic pain spans the full range of sensations and intensity. It can feel tingling, jolting, burning, dull or sharp. The pain may remain constant, or it can come and go, like a migraine that develops without warning.

Unlike acute pain, however, with chronic pain you may not know the reason for the pain. The original injury shows every indication of being healed, yet the pain remains — and may be even more intense.

Chronic pain can also occur without any indication of injury. Years ago, people who complained of pain that had no apparent cause were thought to be imagining the misery or trying to get attention. Doctors now know that's not true. Chronic pain is real.

What causes chronic pain?

Frequently, the cause of chronic pain is not well understood. There may be no evidence of disease or damage to your body tissues that doctors can directly link to the pain.

Sometimes, chronic pain is due to a chronic condition, such as arthritis, which produces painful inflammation in your joints, or fibromyalgia, which causes aching in your muscles.

Occasionally, chronic pain may stem from an accident, infection or surgery that damages a peripheral or spinal nerve. This type of nerve pain that lingers after the original injury heals is called neuropathic (noor-o-PATH-ik) — meaning the damaged nerve, not the original injury, is causing the pain. Neuropathic pain can also result from diseases such as diabetes or alcoholism.

Once damaged, the nerve may send pain messages that are unwarranted. For example, an increased blood sugar level associated with diabetes can damage the small nerves in your hands and feet, leaving you with a painful burning sensation in your fingers and toes.

Little is known about why injured nerves sometimes misfire and send painful messages. However, one reason is that when a nerve cell is destroyed, the severed end of the surviving fiber can sprout a tangle of unorganized nerve fibers (neuroma). This bundle of nerve tissue then starts sending spontaneous pain signals. These fibers also refuse to follow normal checks and balances that control the rest of your nervous system, keeping pain at bay.

Sensitization and pain pathways

It used to be thought that pain transmission pathways in the peripheral nerves, spinal cord and brain were hardwired circuits that simply communicated pain signals from injured or diseased parts of the body to message centers in the brain. But based on recent scientific research, there is new knowledge of how pain transmission actually works and how the conscious experience of pain is created in the brain.

One very important aspect of these new discoveries about pain has to do with a process called sensitization. An introduction to sensitization will help you to understand how your chronic pain can be so severe and why your pain may seem out of proportion to the evidence of injury or disease in the affected body tissues. Sensitization can also explain why specific treatments directed at pain relief may provide only limited benefit.

Although the neurobiology of sensitization is complex, the basic idea behind it is straightforward. When pain signals are transmitted from injured or diseased tissues, these signals can then activate (sensitize) pain circuits in the peripheral nervous system, spinal cord and brain.

The process of sensitization can be compared to the volume control on your stereo, amplifying — and sometimes distorting — the pain message. The result is a painful condition that is severe and out of proportion to the disease or original injury. Sensitization may affect all regions of your nervous system that process pain messages, including the sensing, feeling and thinking centers of the brain. When this occurs, chronic pain may be associated with emotional and psychological suffering.

A good example of sensitization is the problem of phantom limb pain. In this condition, a person can feel intense pain in the place of a missing body part, for example, an arm or a leg that has been amputated because of injury or disease. The difficult-to-treat problem of phantom limb pain is explained by persistent activation (sensitization) in the pain transmission pathways from the site of amputation up to the brain.

There is now scientific evidence to confirm the presence of sensitization in various pain conditions that don't involve amputation. When treatments in such cases are directed at injured or diseased tissues themselves, they have no effect on the sensitized pain pathways in the spinal cord and brain. As a result, little benefit is experienced.

Much scientific research at medical centers around the world is focused on identifying the molecular and cellular processes that cause sensitization. The results of this research are likely to provide new and better treatments for many types of chronic pain.

The challenges of controlling chronic pain

Chronic pain is common. It's estimated that almost half of all Americans experience some form of chronic pain during their lifetime. But coping with the pain is often frustrating.

Pain is a very personal experience. No one except you can completely understand what you're feeling. Persistent pain can also be difficult to treat. Occasionally, surgery can cure or reduce it. And for some types of chronic pain, medication or injections are beneficial. Frequently, though, none of these approaches are very effective.

However, that doesn't mean there isn't any hope. Treatments may not make your pain disappear, but you can learn how to manage your pain and improve your quality of life.

Living well despite chronic pain has a lot to do with your attitude and lifestyle. If you have a negative attitude and view yourself as a victim of your pain, your pain will continue to control you and consume your energy. On the other hand, if you approach your condition with a positive attitude and a willingness to change, you're likely to be successful in coping with your chronic pain.

Key steps to help you live better with chronic pain may include:
- Becoming more physically active
- Organizing your day and performing daily tasks more efficiently
- Practicing techniques that relieve stress
- Identifying your capabilities, not just your limitations
- Understanding and expressing the emotions that pain creates, but not dwelling on the pain itself
- Improving communication with family members and friends
- Weaning yourself from unnecessary medications
- Practicing good health habits, including following a nutritious diet, managing your weight and getting adequate sleep

This book can help you discover what may be contributing to your pain. It also includes strategies and suggestions for how you can make positive life changes. With your doctor, other health care professionals, and your family and friends, you can learn new ways to take control of your pain and your life.

Chapter 2

Do you have
chronic pain?

C hronic pain can affect just about any part of your body, from your head to your toes, from your skin to your internal organs. Arthritis, back pain and headache are the most common types of chronic pain. Your pain may be related to an existing illness or stem from an accident or injury. Perhaps your pain is linked to a condition that doctors don't fully understand. Or maybe it has no apparent cause. In this chapter, some of the more common types of chronic pain are discussed as well as why they occur.

Arthritis

Arthritis means "joint inflammation." Although people often talk about it as one disease, it's not. There are many forms of arthritis. Some forms begin gradually. Others suddenly appear and then disappear, only to return again later. Arthritis can affect any joint in your body and may be triggered by various causes, including an injury, lack of physical activity, natural wear on your joints or genetic disease. The two most common forms of arthritis are osteoarthritis and rheumatoid arthritis.

Osteoarthritis

About half of all arthritis cases are osteoarthritis, and it affects nearly 21 million Americans. This condition results when cartilage that cushions the ends of bones in your joints deteriorates. If the cartilage wears down completely, you may be left with bone rubbing against bone, irritating the joint and producing pain.

Your body tries to repair the damage, but often the repairs are unsuccessful, resulting in growth of new bone along the sides of existing bone. The new bone may produce bony lumps, most noticeably in your hands and feet, and especially in the joints of your fingers and toes. These lumps, called spurs, may or may not produce pain and tenderness.

Osteoarthritis most often develops after age 45 and occurs equally in men and women. It can develop anywhere in your body, but it tends to be most common in your hands and feet and in your neck, lower back, knees and hips. The disease generally is associated with wear on your joints or a specific injury to a joint. But the damage may be related to an imbalance of enzymes in a joint, which causes cartilage to break down.

Initially, arthritis pain may be minor and hurt only when you use the affected joint. In time, the pain can intensify and hurt even when you're not using the joint.

Normal spine

Spine with osteoarthritis

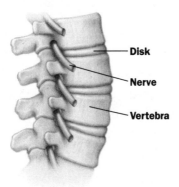 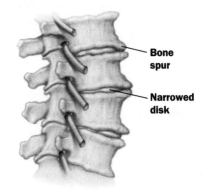

Elastic structures called disks serve as cushions between vertebrae in a normal spine, keeping it flexible. In osteoarthritis, disks narrow, leading to bony lumps along the edges of vertebrae. Pain and stiffness may occur where bone surfaces rub together.

Rheumatoid arthritis

Unlike osteoarthritis, rheumatoid arthritis likely stems from an immune system disorder that causes your immune system to attack the lining in your joints.

White blood cells move into joint tissues,

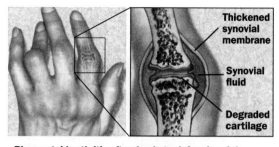

Rheumatoid arthritis often leads to deformity of the fingers and the hand. During flare-ups of the disease, your hand may be painful and weak.

producing inflammation and pain. Swelling of the tissues triggers the release of natural chemicals that can damage cartilage, tendons and ligaments. Gradually, the joint loses its shape. In some cases, the disease destroys the joint.

Rheumatoid arthritis most often affects joints in your wrists, hands, feet and ankles. It can also affect your elbows, shoulders, hips, knees, neck and jaw. In addition to pain and swelling, you may experience stiffness and loss of motion in the joints.

The disease typically develops between ages 20 and 50. An estimated 2 million Americans have rheumatoid arthritis, and roughly twice as many women as men are affected by it.

Back pain

More than 26 million Americans between the ages of 20 and 64 experience frequent back pain, and two thirds of American adults will have back pain during their lifetime. Lower back pain accounts for 3 percent to 6 percent of disability in the population each year.

Most back pain occurs in your lower back (lumbar area), which bears most of your weight. Your lower back also serves as your body's pivot point, allowing you to bend forward and backward and twist sideways.

Acute back pain often stems from an injury or overuse. Usually, there's an accumulation of stress with one particular event causing the pain. But what causes some people to experience lingering, chronic back pain is less clear. This type of pain may be related to one of the following conditions.

Muscle strain and spasm

Muscle strain is a common cause of back pain. It can occur if you lift something too heavy, twist too sharply or stand on your feet too long. Muscle spasm may also occur. Spasm is your back's response to injury, designed to immobilize you and prevent further damage. Any movement of the injured muscles can set off a wave of stabbing pains.

The good news is that about 90 percent of these strains heal within 4 weeks, usually much sooner. The remaining 10 percent take longer to heal. In some cases, the pain never goes away and becomes a chronic problem.

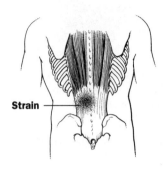

Strain

Your lower back, a pivot point for turning at your waist, is vulnerable to muscle strain.

Sciatica

This condition is named for the sciatic (si-AT-ic) nerve that extends down each leg from your buttock to your heel. Nerve inflammation or compression of a nerve root in your lower back can cause sciatica. You may feel the pain radiating from your back down through your buttock to your lower leg. Tingling, numbness or muscle weakness also can occur.

Another cause of sciatica is related to spasms or tightness in the buttock (gluteal) muscles. This is called piriformis syndrome.

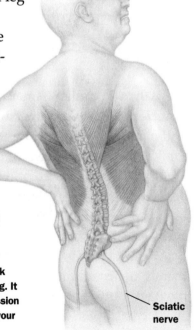

Sciatic nerve

Sciatica is pain that radiates from your back down through your buttock to your lower leg. It may be caused by inflammation or compression of spinal nerve roots which merge to form your sciatic nerve.

Usually, the pain goes away on its own. However, severe nerve compression can cause progressive muscle weakness and continued pain.

Herniated disk

Normal wear and tear or injury can cause a disk between the bones in your back (vertebrae) to bulge or rupture — sometimes called a slipped disk. When the disk ruptures, the rubber-like interior of the disk pokes out from its normal position between your vertebrae.

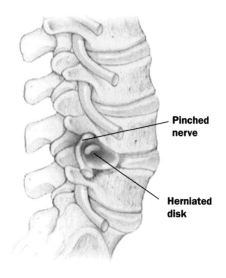

Pinched nerve

Herniated disk

Wear and tear or injury can cause disks to rupture (herniate), creating painful pressure on nerves.

Almost everyone over age 40 has one or more bulging disks, and most aren't bothered by them. But if the bulging material presses against an adjacent nerve, the condition may cause pain.

Generally, the rupture heals over time and the pain goes away. But in some cases, the nerve compression and pain can persist.

Additional causes

Other conditions that may lead to chronic back pain include:
- Joint degeneration from arthritis
- Reduced muscle tone caused by physical inactivity

Complex regional pain syndrome

Minor injury can set this pain off. So can a broken bone, sprain, surgical incision or any number of other injuries — usually to your hand or foot. Before long, you're experiencing a bewildering variety of painful symptoms not only at the injury site but also in adjacent areas.

This condition used to be known as reflex sympathetic dystrophy (RSD) because it was thought to stem from an overreaction of your sympathetic nervous system, part of your autonomic nervous system that controls your heart rate, blood pressure and skin temperature. But now doctors are unsure of its cause. In fact, complex regional pain syndrome — often called CRPS — is one of the least understood forms of chronic pain.

The condition is difficult to diagnose because it's similar to other conditions. However, it typically includes these unique characteristics:

- Pain that lasts longer and more intensely than you would expect from the injury
- Blood flow changes that alter the temperature, color and thickness of skin in the affected area
- Persistent swelling of the affected area

In most cases the pain persists for more than 6 months and in about 25 percent of the cases, for a year or more.

Endometriosis

Endometriosis results when cells from the lining of a woman's uterus (endometrium) migrate through the fallopian tubes and into the abdominal cavity. These cells plant themselves on other structures, such as the pelvic walls and surfaces of the ovaries or fallopian tubes.

Some women with endometriosis experience no pain, but others have frequent pain. The pain may be steady, may worsen during certain times of the menstrual cycle, or it may come and go spontaneously. Often, the pain is described as a pressure-like aching in the lower abdomen, back and rectum that may radiate into the vagina, nearby muscles and thighs.

Other symptoms may include:

- Intense cramping during menstrual periods and pain that extends several days before and after each period
- Deep pelvic pain during intercourse
- Pain during bowel movements or urination

Endometriosis generally doesn't develop until after the onset of menstruation and rarely occurs after menopause.

Fibromyalgia

Fibromyalgia syndrome is a collection of symptoms that includes widespread pain and tenderness. It differs from arthritis in that the pain is in muscles and tissues near the joints instead of in the joints themselves. Also unlike arthritis, it doesn't cause joint or muscle inflammation, nor does it destroy joints or endanger internal organs. It just causes pain.

The main symptom of fibromyalgia is an aching all over. The pain may be a deep ache or a burning sensation. Other signs and symptoms associated with fibromyalgia may include:

- Chronic fatigue
- Difficulty sleeping
- Stiffness
- Headache
- Pain during menstruation
- Dizziness
- Digestive problems
- Numbness
- Tingling
- Sensitivity to weather and temperature changes
- Mood changes

Because these signs and symptoms commonly occur together and no specific cause has been found, fibromyalgia is referred to as a syndrome rather than a disease. In addition, because the symptoms are many and varied and don't follow a consistent pattern, fibromyalgia can be very stressful as well as painful.

Most often, symptoms of fibromyalgia first become noticeable in your 30s. Symptoms may flare up and then subside, but they usually don't disappear completely. Although fibromyalgia tends to stay with you, it isn't progressive or life-threatening.

Doctors aren't sure what causes fibromyalgia. One theory is that certain factors such as stress, poor sleep, physical or emotional trauma or being out-of-shape may trigger the condition. Numerous other possibilities as to its cause also are under study.

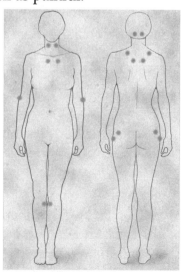

Common locations of tenderness associated with fibromyalgia.

Doctors generally diagnose fibromyalgia based on the typical collection of signs and symptoms and the presence of widespread tenderness, and only after they've tested for and eliminated the possibility of other conditions.

Headache

Of all the pains people experience, headache is the most common complaint. Nearly everyone gets a headache at one time or another.

Headaches can range from fleeting annoyances to those that lay you flat on your back for days and return often enough that they become a chronic problem.

There are several types of headaches. Most fall into one of two categories.

Tension-type headache

This is the most common type of headache. It can range from mild to severe, and can disrupt your daily routine to varying degrees. You may experience a slow-building, dull, tight, pressurized pain that envelopes your forehead, scalp, back of the neck or both sides of your head. Occasionally the pain may be burning or throbbing.

Many cases of tension-type headache appear to result from contraction of the muscles on the outside of your skull. There's some evidence that enlargement of blood vessels in your scalp also may contribute to the pain. Tension-type headaches may be triggered by stressful events such as a demanding job, a bumper-to-bumper commute or an argument with a friend or family member. Staring at a computer screen all day or other prolonged, stressful postures also can produce tension-type headaches. Tension-type headaches can become a chronic problem.

Migraine headache

More than 25 million Americans experience a more painful variety of headache known as migraine. This type of headache not only gets your attention but also can put your life on hold.

Migraines generally produce throbbing pain on one side of your head — often your temple or forehead. Bright lights and loud noises

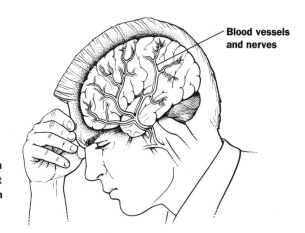

Blood vessels
and nerves

Migraines appear to stem from an
imbalance of brain chemicals that
causes blood vessels in your brain
to swell and signal pain.

may intensify the pain, and you may become nauseated and vomit. The pain can range from moderate to severe. Most migraines develop for only a few hours before peaking and slowly subsiding.

Migraines were once thought to be chiefly related to blood circulation. During a migraine attack, blood vessels in your brain, neck and scalp tighten, reducing blood flow to your brain. This tightening is followed by expansion of the vessels to larger than their normal size, producing swelling and pain.

Researchers now believe these changes are a result of, and not the cause of, migraines. A more likely cause is an imbalance of brain chemicals. Several chemicals may be related in some way to the development of migraines, including the brain chemical serotonin (ser-o-TOE-nin). During a headache, serotonin levels generally drop.

About 10 percent of people with recurrent migraines get warning symptoms of an impending headache. These signals, called auras, often involve tingling sensations or visual distortions, such as blurred vision or zigzagging lights. They generally last less than an hour, often just 10 to 30 minutes.

Migraines appear to be hereditary. They may be triggered by several factors:

Hormone fluctuations. Three times more women than men are affected by migraines. About 15 percent of women who get migraines say they occur only before, during or right after their periods. Estrogen found in birth control pills and in hormone therapy also may trigger migraine attacks in some women. For other women, their migraines diminish when taking estrogen.

Diet. Between 8 percent and 25 percent of people with migraines point to a particular food as a trigger for their attacks. The most common culprits are alcohol (especially red wine and beer), aged cheeses, chocolate, caffeine, monosodium glutamate (MSG) and fermented, pickled or marinated foods. In addition, going too long without eating and caffeine withdrawal also can cause migraines.

Environment. Many people cite bright light, strong odors or changes in weather conditions as triggers for migraines.

Lifestyle. Daily stress can trigger a migraine. Migraines may also result from poor or changing sleep patterns, extreme fatigue and stress and relief from stress.

Medications. Several medications may trigger a migraine in people who are susceptible to the headaches. They include certain high blood pressure medications, birth control pills and hormone therapy. Frequent use of a pain medication also may cause a migraine when the dose wears off. This is called a rebound withdrawal headache.

Interstitial cystitis

This painful bladder condition affects mainly women. It results from chronic inflammation of your bladder wall. What causes it to develop is unknown.

Symptoms include pressure, pain and tenderness around the bladder, a frequent need to urinate and backaches. In some people, the pain can be so severe that they have trouble riding in a car or even sitting at a desk.

The condition often mimics symptoms of a urinary tract infection, but urine tests don't detect any bacteria and antibiotics don't relieve the pain.

Irritable bowel syndrome

Irritable bowel syndrome (IBS) — also referred to as functional bowel disorder — is a complex disorder in your lower intestinal tract that causes pain, bloating, gas and recurrent bouts of diarrhea or constipation. It's a common gastrointestinal disorder and a frequent reason people see a doctor. Fortunately, IBS causes no structural damage to the bowel.

The pain accompanying this condition often occurs below the navel and can be dull and aching or sharp and sudden. The condition may stem from disturbances in the nerves that control sensation or muscle contractions in your bowel. Your central nervous system or hormonal changes also may play a role. Hormone fluctuations help explain why some women's symptoms are worse before or during menstruation.

Some evidence shows that people with IBS have intestines that react more strongly to stress, activity or diet than do those in people without the condition. There's little evidence that IBS results from particular foods. However, in some cases, fatty foods, beans and other gas-producing foods, alcohol, caffeine and excess dietary fiber may make symptoms worse.

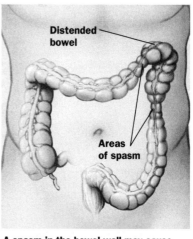

A spasm in the bowel wall may cause abdominal pain and other unpleasant symptoms commonly associated with irritable bowel syndrome.

Mouth, jaw and face pain

Some people experience chronic pain in their mouth, jaws and face (orofacial pain). Often, this pain is the result of dental problems, such as cavities or gum disease. But sometimes it can stem from other orofacial conditions.

Burning mouth syndrome

With burning mouth syndrome (BMS), you may have a burning sensation on your tongue or lips, or more widespread burning that involves your entire mouth. It's estimated that BMS affects up to 5 percent of adults in the United States — women seven times more often than men. Causes include chronic infections, reflux of stomach acid, blood diseases, hormone imbalances and medication side effects.

Trigeminal neuralgia

Also known as tic douloureux (doo-loo-ROO), this pain can develop when a blood vessel comes in contact with the trigeminal (tri-JEM-ih-nul) nerve, putting pressure on the nerve. The trigeminal nerve branches throughout your face and controls facial sensations and some muscles involved in chewing.

Trigeminal neuralgia can cause an electric shock-like pain on one side of your face and may cause you to wince as though you've been hit in the face. Jolts of pain may persist from a few seconds to 1 to 2 minutes, usually returning many times a day.

Most trigeminal neuralgia pain occurs spontaneously, but it's sometimes triggered by touching your face, eating, talking, brushing your teeth or a breeze on your face.

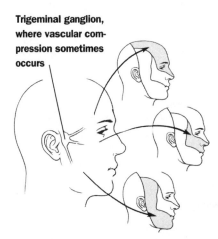

Trigeminal ganglion, where vascular compression sometimes occurs

If you have trigeminal neuralgia, pain may occur in areas supplied by one of the three branches of the trigeminal (fifth cranial) nerve.

Temporomandibular disorders

The temporomandibular joints, located on each side of your face, connect your jaw to your skull. Temporomandibular joint disorders refer to a group of symptoms affecting these joints and their attached muscles. A common symptom is pain in your jaw, face, neck or ear.

Other signs and symptoms may include headaches, jaw locking or catching, and pops or clicks in your jaw during normal use.

There are several theories regarding the causes of these disorders.

Your temporomandibular joint is a hinged joint situated on each side of your head where the lower jawbone (mandible) connects with the temporal bone of your skull. Inflammation, injury or dislocation of this joint may cause pain.

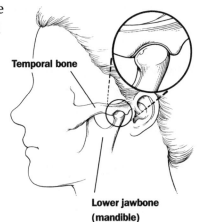

Temporal bone

Lower jawbone (mandible)

They include trauma to the joints, degeneration of the joints and disturbance of the muscles surrounding the joints.

Other causes
Orofacial pain can also occur for other reasons that aren't well understood — and that are difficult to diagnose. Many times, the pain develops after dental treatment or a facial injury. It may be a constant aching or burning. Or it may come in the form of frequent shocks. Nerve damage in a tooth and damage to nerves in your face are possible causes. Postherpetic neuralgia (see page 28) is also a common cause of facial pain.

Neck pain

Similar to back pain, an injury or poor posture can strain muscles, ligaments or tendons in your neck, producing inflammation and pain. Most of the time the pain lasts for just a few days or weeks. Occasionally, it can become chronic.

Neck pain may also stem from a herniated disk or degeneration of joints in your upper spine as a result of osteoarthritis. Instead of sliding across each other smoothly, bony surfaces in your neck grate or rub on each other, causing stiffness and pain.

Often, one pain leads to another. You automatically tense your neck muscles to prevent further movement in a sore spot. The tension produces pain and may also trigger a painful muscle spasm.

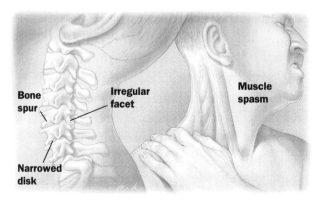

Bone spur

Irregular facet

Muscle spasm

Narrowed disk

Disks between bones in your neck can thin and lose elasticity. Bony outgrowths (spurs) may form. As joints rub together with greater-than-normal force, surfaces where they meet become irregular. Pain may result.

Overuse strain injuries

These injuries result from overuse of your muscles and tendons — mainly those in your hands, wrists and arms. The most noticeable symptom is pain. But an overuse injury can also cause tingling, weakness, numbness, swelling and stiffness.

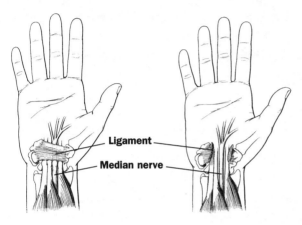

Ligament

Median nerve

A narrow tunnel through your wrist (the carpal tunnel) protects your median nerve, which provides sensation to your fingers. When swelling occurs in the tunnel, the median nerve can become compressed, producing pain.

Computer users, assembly line employees and meat cutters are among those commonly affected by an overuse injury. But it can occur in anyone who uses repeated motions in his or her daily activities.

Carpal tunnel syndrome is the most recognized overuse injury. It results from constant strain on your wrist, which can inflame the tendons below your carpal ligament, the ligament that stretches across the palm side of your wrist. When the tendons swell, they press against a nearby nerve located beneath your carpal ligament, producing pain. Because the nerve runs up your arm all the way to your neck, you might feel pain anywhere along that pathway.

Most often, the result is intermittent numbness, tingling or pain starting in your wrist and moving down into your thumb and first two or three fingers. Some people find their symptoms are worse at night because of the position of their wrist or arm while sleeping. The position of your wrists when holding a book or driving a car may also bring on symptoms.

Pelvic pain

One in seven women experience some form of chronic pelvic pain (CPP), and it accounts for 10 percent to 20 percent of office visits to a gynecologist. No physical cause may be found for CPP, but here are some known causes:

- Pelvic floor tension myalgia is due to spasms of the pelvic floor muscles, which loop around the rectum and attach to the front of the pelvis.
- Chronic pelvic inflammatory disease (PID) can occur if a long-term infection causes your fallopian tubes to scar and stick to your ovaries.
- Pelvic congestion syndrome may be caused by varicose-type veins around your ovaries. These veins may lead to blood pooling in the ovaries and pelvic area.
- Ovarian remnant occurs when small pieces of ovary left behind after a hysterectomy develop into tiny, painful cysts.
- Fibroids are noncancerous uterine growths that rarely cause pain until they disintegrate. However, they can cause pressure or a feeling of heaviness in your lower abdomen.

Peripheral neuropathy

This nerve-related condition most often affects your hands and feet, causing a tingling pain that can be accompanied by numbness. In some cases, the pain can also be shooting or burning.

Peripheral neuropathy can result from many causes, such as the side effects of medications — including some chemotherapy drugs — as well as infection or vitamin deficiencies. The most common causes are diabetes, alcoholism, autoimmune diseases such as rheumatoid arthritis or lupus, and hereditary neuropathies. There are also times when the cause of peripheral neuropathy is unclear.

The condition usually starts with a tingling sensation in your toes or the balls of your feet that spreads upward. Occasionally, it begins in your hands and extends up your arms. Numbness and weakness may follow, but the amount of pain doesn't necessarily correlate with other symptoms. Your skin also may become highly sensitive.

Postherpetic neuralgia

Postherpetic neuralgia (post-her-PET-ic noo-RAL-jah) refers to nerve damage that can occur as a result of shingles. Shingles (herpes zoster) is caused by a reactivation of the chickenpox virus in nerve tissues. The damaged fibers aren't able to send normal pain messages. Instead, the messages become distorted and exaggerated, producing unrelenting, and often severe, pain.

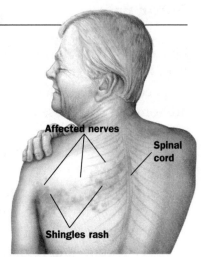

Shingles rash is associated with an inflammation of nerves beneath the skin. Damage to the nerves may produce postherpetic neuralgia.

Pain associated with acute shingles can take different forms, including burning, sharp and jabbing, or deep and aching. Your skin also may become hypersensitive. The slightest touch of clothing or even a change in temperature can produce a flare of pain.

Postherpetic neuralgia affects half the people older than age 60 with shingles and 75 percent of people older than age 70 with shingles. For many people, the condition gradually disappears on its own, but this can take months to several years.

Unknown causes

Sometimes, chronic pain develops for no apparent reason. Despite repeated tests, your doctor isn't able to link it to an identifiable physical cause or condition. This doesn't mean that the pain is imagined. It simply means that your pain may be associated with factors that are difficult to diagnose.

Your health is also affected by the interaction of your mind and body. For some people, psychological issues can play a major role in chronic pain. For example, people who've endured sexual abuse or other kinds of physical abuse appear to have a greater risk of developing chronic pelvic or abdominal pain. It's unknown whether the pain is the result of physical injuries or if it stems from emotional scars or stress. It may be due to a combination of factors.

Chapter 3

Cycles of chronic pain

People living with chronic pain often compare their lives to a roller coaster ride. There are good days when they feel uplifted and in control, followed by bad days when their mood sinks and they feel helpless. Rarely does pain stay at an even level. It fluctuates. Pain also doesn't have any boundaries. When a part of you is in pain, your whole body reacts.

As you try to understand, accept and manage your condition, your behavior and emotions may go through a series of ups and downs. This is especially true if you have debilitating pain. Often, these behavioral and emotional changes follow a predictable pattern.

Behavioral cycle

One of the first noticeable effects of chronic pain is the change it brings in your day-to-day activities. Regular tasks often become more difficult or impossible.

The following scenario — outlined in stages — is an example of how chronic pain often works and how it can easily alter your routine and behavior.

Stage 1: Decrease in activity

Because of your pain, just getting the yard rake down from its hook in the garage — much less raking the entire yard — seems like too big a chore.

So instead, you let the leaves fall. But every time you pass by a window, you're reminded of what you can't do.

You could hire someone to rake the yard, but that would cost money. You could have your family do it, but they might feel resentful that you're not out helping them. Plus, you don't like the idea of watching others take over your responsibilities.

So you wait for a day when you feel better.

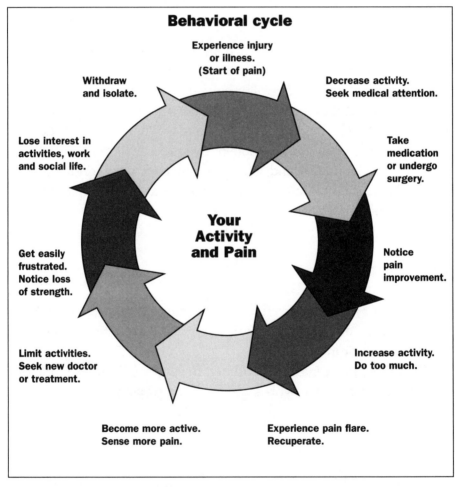

Uncontrolled chronic pain commonly causes this pattern of behavior, beginning at the top of the circle and moving clockwise.

Stage 2: Increase in activity

When the day arrives that you feel better, you rake the yard. But you also run errands, clean the garage and go out to dinner with friends.

You put in a day best fit for a superhero. But as long as you're feeling well, why not catch up on all those things you've been neglecting?

Stage 3: More pain, less activity

The next day, you can hardly move. You feel worse than you did before your superheroic day. You chastise yourself for trying to do too much at one time and spend the next few days resting and trying to recuperate.

Eventually, you begin to feel better. But as you start to become more active, your pain worsens. Thinking that the only way to control your pain is to limit all physical activity, you turn over many of your daily chores to family members or friends and spend more time in bed or on the couch.

Meanwhile, more leaves fall, friends keep calling, and you don't feel up to doing anything.

Stage 4: Loss of strength and physical deconditioning

The time you spend lying around is making you tired, weak and less able to finish up the yardwork. Because of your long stretch of inactivity, your stamina is leaving you. You get fatigued easily. Even the thought of physical labor is daunting.

Stage 5: Withdrawal and isolation

You find yourself spending more time alone and less time with those who care about you. Because you've stopped going out with your friends, they've stopped calling. They figure that you'd just turn them down anyway, so why bother?

Your family has become accustomed to doing things without you. They now rake the yard without your help and they've also started going out to dinner and attending social events without you. They think they're accommodating you by not forcing you to go.

You retreat even further from your family, friends and favorite activities. Eventually, a day comes when you begin to feel a little better. It's followed by another good day, and you feel optimistic that your condition may finally be improving. But once again, your pain flares, and the cycle repeats itself.

Communicating your pain

When you're in pain, others can often tell it by your actions. These actions, called pain behaviors, refer to the things you do or say that lets people know you're experiencing pain. They're ways of calling attention to your pain — either consciously or unconsciously.

Pain behaviors are a natural response to pain. During an initial period of acute pain, they may help reduce your pain. But over time they become ineffective. For people with chronic pain, pain behaviors often become a habit.

Common pain behaviors include:

- Limping
- Crying
- Groaning
- Grimacing
- Limiting activity
- Staying in bed
- Using protective posture
- Talking about pain, surgery or bodily functions
- Withdrawing from others

People around you generally react in one of two ways to pain behaviors: They become annoyed by them — "Not this again" — or they become overly attentive to the behaviors — "Here, let me do that." Either response creates an unequal relationship in which people tend to focus more on your illness rather than on the healthier aspects of your life.

Pain behaviors also consume a lot of energy that could be channeled into other, more productive ventures, such as taking steps to manage your pain.

Emotional cycle

Just as your behavior fluctuates when you're in pain, so do your emotions. Often, the two go hand in hand — the more you're able to do, the better your mood, and the less you're able to do, the worse your mood. Like your behaviors, your emotions also tend to follow a cyclic pattern.

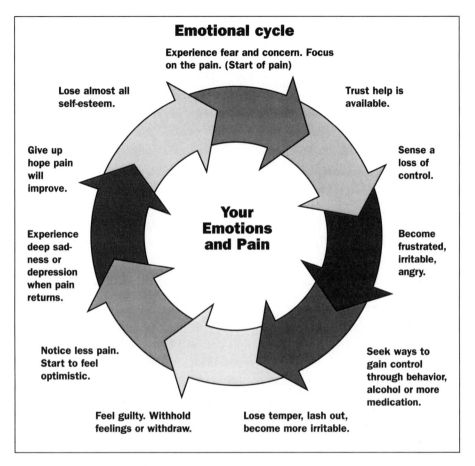

Emotional cycle

Experience fear and concern. Focus on the pain. (Start of pain)

Trust help is available.

Lose almost all self-esteem.

Sense a loss of control.

Give up hope pain will improve.

Your Emotions and Pain

Become frustrated, irritable, angry.

Experience deep sadness or depression when pain returns.

Notice less pain. Start to feel optimistic.

Seek ways to gain control through behavior, alcohol or more medication.

Feel guilty. Withhold feelings or withdraw.

Lose temper, lash out, become more irritable.

Uncontrolled chronic pain commonly causes this pattern of emotions, beginning at the top of the circle and moving clockwise.

Stage 1: Fear and concern

When you first experience your pain, you're fearful and concerned. You worry that your pain may be a symptom of a disabling or serious disease. Your pain becomes the focus of your attention. The more you worry about it, the worse it seems to get, and in turn, the harder it is to ignore.

Stage 2: Hope and promise

When you finally learn what's triggering your pain, your fear and concern are replaced with hope that your doctor will be able to make the pain disappear and your life will soon return to normal. If your doctor isn't able to find a cause, at least knowing that your pain isn't a symptom of a life-threatening condition makes you feel better.

You think that curing your pain is a reasonable request. In today's society, when something breaks we expect someone to fix it. But repairing your body is far more complicated than fixing your car or a household appliance. When the pain continues to linger despite repeated trips to various doctors, your hope starts to diminish.

Stage 3: Anger and frustration

You become dejected and depressed over the state of your life. This is the stage when you ask, "Why me?" and "What did I do to deserve this?" On some level, you may know that the pain isn't a punishment. But, still, you feel as if you've done something wrong, and now you're paying the price.

You may also find it easy to vent your frustration on others — your doctors, your insurance representatives and even your own family and friends. But it's displaced anger. What's upsetting you may be the long waits at your doctor's office, the bill at the end of each visit, increased dependence on others, a sense of loss of control or, perhaps most of all, no relief from your pain.

As your life feels less and less your own, you may seek to gain control in other, destructive ways, such as increasing pain medication on your own, drinking too much alcohol or illicitly using drugs. You may become more irritable with the people who are trying their best to help you.

Stage 4: Guilt and withdrawal

You feel guilty over the things you've said and done. Instead of communicating this guilt, you withdraw from people so that you won't take your anger out on them.

You also feel guilty because you aren't able to do your full share anymore. Your spouse or children have taken over some of your duties, such as parenting responsibilities, cleaning the house or raking the yard. At work, you can't keep up your normal pace and your co-workers are having to lend you a hand. Instead of venting your frustrations, you may start to withhold your emotions and keep them bottled up inside.

Stage 5: Renewed hope, followed by depression

Gradually, or perhaps rather suddenly, you feel better. You're optimistic that your condition is finally improving or the new treatment you're trying is working. Excitedly, you start getting back into your old routine. But after a time, the pain returns and you become deeply disappointed and lose all hope of recovery. You feel depressed and find that you can hardly make it out of bed in the morning. Things that used to matter to you, such as your appearance or attending family or social activities, don't seem important.

You begin to feel as though you're no longer loved or needed, and your self-esteem hits an all-time low. You may even begin to wonder if you're deserving of love and attention. As you draw deeper inside yourself, your pain becomes the focus of all of your attention. Fear, isolation and depression, coupled with days of nothing to do, make the pain feel even worse. The severity of your pain finally forces you to look for other forms of treatment, setting you up for a repeat of the cycle.

Overachiever's curse

Living with chronic pain isn't easy. But it can be especially difficult if you've prided yourself on being a perfectionist or always on the go.

If you're the sort of person who gets things done and is always called on to complete a project on time, make the cookies for the bake sale or coach the Little League team, being unable to do your part because of your pain can be devastating.

When chronic pain hits, an overachiever often has to settle for being just like everyone else. This causes some people to fall victim to all-or-nothing thinking. If they can't head the committee, they don't even want to be involved. They completely dismiss themselves from their normal activities and become withdrawn and depressed.

Your family's responses

Your pain, and how you react to it, also affects your family. Their responses to your behavior and emotions can take on parallel cycles of their own.

Family behaviors

When chronic pain first becomes a problem, family members generally show a great deal of support. They're often increasingly attentive to you, making sure you're as comfortable as possible. They do more tasks around the house so that you can relax and "get better."

Family members also become vigilant in assessing your pain and keeping track of the activities that seem to make it better or worse. They observe and monitor you closely, in an attempt to help lessen your pain and help your doctor make a diagnosis.

When your pain doesn't improve, your family's patience may start to wear thin. At this stage, they begin to resent the extra burden they've been handed. And though most family members realize that it's not your fault, it becomes difficult to separate the person from the pain. They may begin to withdraw and pay less attention to you.

Family emotions

Family members often go through the very same emotions you do. Initially, they fear the cause of your pain. Later, when your treatment doesn't seem to be working and they're shouldering more responsibilities, they become angry and begin to ask, "Why me?" — or more appropriately, "Why us?"

Just as you do, family members often feel a loss of control over their daily life and normal routine. This frustration can lead them to withhold affection because they're angry at the situation facing them. They may unintentionally take this anger out on you.

They feel bad about being angry with you and, in turn, start to feel bad about themselves and how they're acting. "I'm not a good person" and "I should be able to handle this" are common thoughts. Their guilt often leads to increased attentiveness and care, beginning the emotional cycle again.

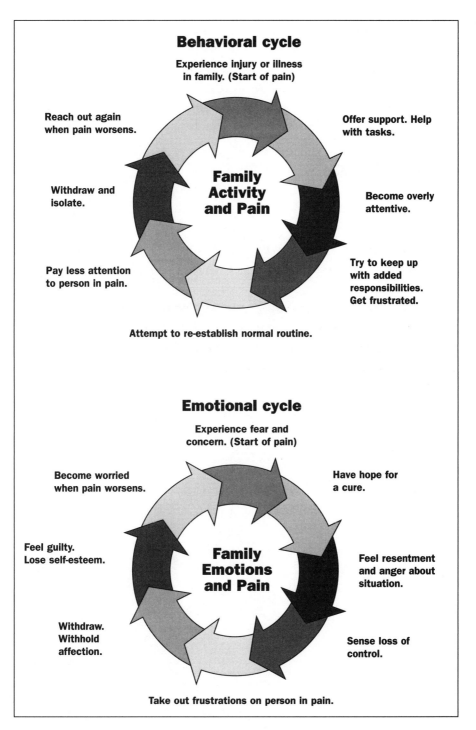

Behavioral cycle

Experience injury or illness
in family. (Start of pain)

Reach out again
when pain worsens.

Offer support. Help
with tasks.

**Family
Activity
and Pain**

Withdraw and
isolate.

Become overly
attentive.

Pay less attention
to person in pain.

Try to keep up
with added
responsibilities.
Get frustrated.

Attempt to re-establish normal routine.

Emotional cycle

Experience fear and
concern. (Start of pain)

Become worried
when pain worsens.

Have hope for
a cure.

**Family
Emotions
and Pain**

Feel guilty.
Lose self-esteem.

Feel resentment
and anger about
situation.

Withdraw.
Withhold
affection.

Sense loss of
control.

Take out frustrations on person in pain.

Family members commonly experience patterns of behavior and emotion that are similar to those
of the person in pain.

Unfortunately, even though you and your family share common feelings, you may find these feelings difficult to talk about. Your family members fear it will sound as if they're blaming you for your pain. They also don't want to come across as being selfish and inconsiderate. You have many of the same fears. The silence, however, often brings more resentment and frustration.

Breaking the cycles

You may think that the cycles of chronic pain will never end. But you can break free of them. The downward spiral that often accompanies chronic pain occurs when all of your attention is focused on your pain. To reduce your pain, you change your life, often in ways you don't like.

By learning how to manage your pain so that it's no longer the focus of your attention, you can concentrate on the things that give you pleasure and satisfaction. This renewed feeling of control over your life will help you end the pain cycles.

Chapter 4

Costs of chronic pain

N ot everyone experiences the rippling effects of chronic pain. Some people can live with their pain without it taking a toll on their daily lives and overall health. Others aren't as lucky. If you're suffering significantly because of your pain, you're not alone.

This chapter details the personal and economic costs associated with chronic pain. It's not an upbeat discussion. But the good news is that the story doesn't end here. This book is about improving your quality of life, despite your pain. The chapters that follow outline what you can do to help minimize these personal and economic costs and, in some cases, avoid them.

Physical deconditioning

You know that you need regular physical activity to stay healthy. But when you're in pain, you don't feel like being active. Like many people, you may have started an exercise routine. But you did too much the first day. The next day you felt so much worse that the thought of exercising again was more than you could handle.

Inactivity can lead to increased body fat. In addition to weight gain, a higher proportion of body fat increases your risk of cardio-vascular disease and diabetes. Inactivity can also weaken your bones and lead to a higher risk of osteoporosis. As your body becomes more deconditioned, you may begin to feel as though you may never be healthy again.

For more on proper exercise, see Chapter 10.

Loss of sleep

Chronic pain reduces restful sleep. According to a Gallup poll sponsored by the National Sleep Foundation, 62 percent of people with chronic pain reported awakening too early because of their pain and were unable to fall back to sleep.

In addition to the direct effect of pain on sleep, other factors associated with chronic pain can indirectly influence how much and how well you rest:

Lack of physical activity. Inactivity makes it more difficult for you to relax and sleep well.

Excessive alcohol. Drinking too much alcohol reduces restorative sleep by interfering with your brain's ability to produce adequate periods of deep sleep.

Medications. Some pain medications can stimulate your nervous system, so you don't feel tired.

When you don't get adequate sleep, you lack energy, are more easily irritated and aren't able to cope as well with pain and stress. Regular or extended bouts of sleeplessness can also wear on your health. Your body needs restorative sleep to keep all of its systems working properly.

For more information, see "Getting a good night's sleep" on page 155.

Emotional upheaval

Pain can play havoc with your emotions. One minute you may feel fine, the next your world may feel as though it's been torn apart. For some people, that's a specific event. An accident or fall can change your life in an instant. For others, the development of chronic pain is a more gradual process. In either case, the pain has divided your life into two distinct parts — life as you knew it before the pain and life as you now know it afterward.

In your new life, you may feel powerless and trapped. Your emotions may range from fear and frustration to anger and apathy. Dealing with these emotions is often difficult. As you long for life before the pain, the more frustrated or angry you become.

When you're in pain, your sense of security also may disappear. What if I lose my job? Will my family understand? What do my friends think of me? The more anxious you become about your situation, the more stressed you feel. For more on dealing with your emotions, see Chapter 12.

Depression

Depression and chronic pain often go hand in hand. Emotional strain, combined with persistent pain, creates a sinkhole that can be difficult to escape. Studies indicate that up to half the people with chronic pain experience a form of depression.

It's natural to experience some discouragement when chronic pain first develops or for short periods afterward. Your pain itself may also cause symptoms associated with depression, such as slowed movements or loss of energy. But if your symptoms linger for several months or they become severe, you may be experiencing depression.

A person with depression may have some, most or all of these symptoms:
- Lasting sadness
- Loss of interest or pleasure in most activities
- Irritability and mood swings
- Change in appetite and weight (gain or loss)
- Recurrent early awakening or other changes in sleep patterns
- Feelings of restlessness
- Feelings of hopelessness or helplessness
- Extreme fatigue, loss of energy or slowed movements
- Continual negative view of others and the world

- Feelings of worthlessness or inappropriate feelings of guilt
- Neglect of personal responsibilities and care
- Decreased concentration, attention and memory
- Decreased sex drive
- Increased focus on physical complaints
- Thoughts of death or suicide

The fundamental causes of depression aren't fully understood, but psychological and biological factors are both clearly important. Genetic factors, imbalances in certain body or brain chemicals or abnormal sleep behaviors also may give rise to depression. In addition, living with chronic pain and having to give up enjoyable and pleasurable activities may lead to depression.

Regardless of the cause, depression is a complex condition that can make your pain feel worse. That's because it's difficult to separate your mood from your pain intensity. People who are depressed often report stronger, longer-lasting and more severe pain than do people who aren't depressed.

Depression makes pain worse and should be treated. Treating depression can result in less pain or pain that's easier to manage. With treatment, up to 80 percent of people with depression show some improvement, usually in a matter of weeks. However, many people don't receive treatment because they're unaware of their condition or they don't view depression as an illness. Instead, they think that they can handle the condition on their own. To learn about medications that are used to treat depression, see "Medications for associated symptoms" on page 60.

Difficulties at work

At first, your employer may have been sympathetic to you. Perhaps your boss made your workload lighter to accommodate you, or your co-workers pitched in to help you out. But, often, as the pain progresses, things change.

Troubles with a boss or lack of understanding from co-workers can make work a stressful place. This only adds to the pain. If you're having trouble keeping up, you may also fear that you'll lose your job.

Often, the result is some difficult decisions. Options to control your pain and stress may include requesting a shorter workday or changing jobs. But that may not be possible or may involve some unacceptable compromises. For example, another, less stressful position may not offer a comparable salary or insurance benefits.

Financial strain

Medical bills, medications and lost days of work can strain your finances. If your pain has forced you to change or quit your job, your current income may not be sufficient to meet your expenses. To make up for the drop in income, perhaps your spouse has found a new job or is working additional hours.

Some people reach a point where they need to see a financial consultant or move to a less expensive home to avoid bankruptcy. All of these financial worries can compound your pain and further drain your sense of self-esteem.

Damaged relationships

People who were once supportive and always offering to lend a hand may not be around as much. They've gone on with their lives and seem to have less time for you.

Family relationships also seem strained. Even though your family knows you're not to blame, they're frustrated for the way your pain has changed your life and theirs.

Communication in general may be difficult. You get irritated easily and find yourself taking out your emotions on those closest to you. Or to the contrary, you withdraw and don't share your thoughts or feelings at all.

Your pain may also be straining your sexual relationship. Some people experience sexual difficulties due to pain, stress or medications. Others avoid intimacy and sexual intercourse because they no longer feel sexually attractive or they fear intercourse will increase their pain. For more on managing your relationships, see Chapter 14.

Chemical dependency

Reliance on medications can be a troublesome side effect of chronic pain. Signs that medication use may be a problem include:
- A preoccupation with taking medications
- Taking more medication than prescribed
- Use of more than one physician or pharmacy to get medication
- Hiding medications or being secretive about their use
- Using someone else's medication
- Frequent use of an emergency room to get medication
- Drowsiness or periods when you can't recall events

Some people also turn to alcohol or illegal drug use to find relief from their pain and pressures. This can lead to chemical dependency as well. Plus, when you combine prescription medications with other drugs, including alcohol, you increase your risk for dangerous side effects. For more on the stages of drug dependence, see "Getting clear about the risk of addiction" on page 56.

Side effects of dependency
Serious problems can develop when drugs are misused:

Impaired mental functioning. This includes drowsiness, an inability to concentrate and impaired memory.

Physical complications. Damage may occur to many of your organs, including your liver, kidneys and brain.

Emotional distress. You may regularly experience feelings of anxiety, irritability, apathy and depression.

Taking one step at a time

Overcoming the costs of your pain may seem daunting. But remember that the problems that chronic pain can produce are often linked. And even a few small steps can bring noticeable results. For example, making an effort to reduce daily stress can have a positive effect on your physical health, sleep, work, personal relationships, finances and depression. As you begin to see improvements, the challenges ahead may seem less troubling.

Part 2

Treating chronic pain

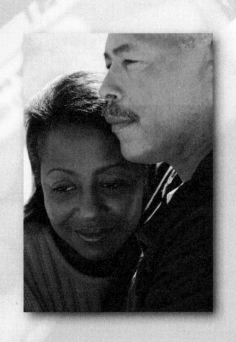

Chapter 5

What about medication?

A dvances in medicine have created a wide range of options for treating chronic pain. One is medication. When used appropriately, medications can help to reduce pain with limited side effects for some people. They can also help control a temporary flare in your pain. In addition, medications may help to treat other conditions that can accompany chronic pain, such as depression and insomnia.

This chapter examines the role of medications in treating chronic pain and offers suggestions for getting the most from your medications. You'll also find information about specific medications, including:

- Simple analgesics
- Opioids (narcotics)
- Topical medications
- Medications that support pain treatment
- Medications for associated symptoms
- Medications for specific pain conditions

Choosing pain medication

The role of medications in treating chronic pain is complex and sometimes controversial. There are many kinds of medications, and doctors have varying opinions about them and how they should be used.

In part, the controversy results from the very nature of chronic
pain. Treating this kind of pain can be more difficult than treating
acute pain, which is often a short-term condition with a clear cause.

To prescribe medications that effectively help with chronic pain,
your doctor has to balance a number of factors. Knowing about
these factors can help you understand your treatment plan:

- **Rehabilitation.** Treatment of chronic pain should not simply
  aim to suppress symptoms. Instead, the larger goal is to help
  you lead a full, active life. Pain medication may help you
  return to a full work schedule, sustain relationships and carry
  out other tasks of daily life.
- **Efficacy.** This term refers to the power of a medication to produce desired results — in this case, a reduction in the level of
  pain. Higher doses of a medication may not increase its efficacy. In fact, a higher dose may increase the risk of side effects.
- **Safety.** Pain medications can cause side effects such as stomach bleeding and liver damage. Over the short term, you may
  find that you can tolerate side effects. However, when medication is used for weeks or months, the risk of side effects becomes a larger issue.
- **Interactions.** Your doctor will try to avoid drug combinations
  that cause unsafe interactions — unwanted effects that can
  occur when some drugs are taken together. Equally important
  is preventing drug-disease interactions — prescribing a drug
  for chronic pain that may worsen another condition, such as
  diabetes. Finally, interactions with over-the-counter medications, alcohol and certain foods also may cause problems.
- **Allergies.** An allergy to one pain medication may eliminate an
  entire class of drugs that could be used in your treatment.
- **Life setting.** To understand this factor, compare two people.
  One is an older adult who has high levels of pain due to an
  end-stage cancer. Another is a middle-aged person with chronic

back pain who still maintains a full work and family life. The person with cancer may have a treatment plan that calls for higher doses of medication to deliver immediate pain relief. The second person may need to balance dosage and pain relief with safety and ability to function in daily life.

- **Placebo effects.** If you try a new pain medication, both you and your doctor may have high hopes for positive results. And, in fact, you might feel better at first, even though the new medication has no specific advantage over a previously used medication. This is the placebo effect, and it can complicate treatment for chronic pain.

- **Practical issues.** You and your doctor also need to consider the cost of your medication and the challenges of sticking to a medication schedule. Some pain medications are short acting and must be taken several times a day. Other medications have longer-lasting effects and can be taken less often.

In light of all these factors, your doctor will tailor your medication to your specific needs and circumstances, applying the concept of hierarchical treatment. This means that your treatment often takes place in stages. You'll probably begin with fewer medications in lower doses with fewer potential side effects. You and your doctor will judge how well this approach works before trying stronger medications, adding to the number of medications, increasing doses or risking more side effects.

Remember that medication is usually just one option in a full treatment plan. Your plan might also include nerve blocks, physical therapy, counseling and lifestyle changes. Some people with chronic pain find that these other options help them reduce or eliminate the need for pain medication.

Getting the most from your medications

According to the Agency for Healthcare Research and Quality, the single most important thing you can do to get the most from your medication is to take an active role in your health care. Use the following steps to increase the safety and efficacy of your medications.

Share information

To create an effective treatment plan, your doctor needs to know exactly which medications you use. Keep an up-to-date list of all of your medications — including what you take to relieve pain — or keep your medications in their original containers and bring them along when you go to the doctor. Include prescription and over-the-counter (OTC) medications, dietary supplements and herbs.

Share these key details about your medications:

- **Name of medication.** To avoid confusion, remember that medications have both generic and brand names.
- **Dosage.** This includes the amount of medication you take at one time and how often you take the medication.
- **Purpose.** Try to remember why you began the medication. For example, was the medication prescribed to treat your pain — or to treat a condition associated with chronic pain, such as insomnia?
- **How you take the medication.** For instance, do you take the medication with or without food? Do you take it just before going to bed or earlier in the day?
- **Results.** Are you feeling any unexpected side effects from the medication? How well do you think the medication is working overall?
- **Other health conditions.** If you're allergic to certain medications or think you might be pregnant, be sure to tell your doctor. Also mention any other illnesses or conditions you have, particularly kidney or liver disease.

Seek information

To aid your memory, keep and read the printed materials that come with your medications. These materials offer general, introductory information. Ask your pharmacist and doctor for information that's specific to you. Find out exactly why you're taking the medication and what results you can expect.

Stick to your plan

It's important that you take medication exactly as prescribed. If you stop taking medication before your prescription ends, you could undermine your treatment results. The same thing can happen if you cut down on medication without consulting your doctor or if you take additional medications without your doctor's knowledge.

If you do depart from your medication plan, tell your doctor. Speaking candidly about how you actually use medications will help your doctor fine-tune your prescriptions.

Speak up

Your mental and physical state can change with time. Medication that worked well for you several months or years ago could have different effects on you today. Sometimes doses need to be changed or the whole treatment plan needs to be adjusted.

To stay on top of your condition, carefully observe day-to-day changes in your health and report those changes. In addition, keep a list of questions to ask your doctor and pharmacist.

Don't be afraid to contact your doctor with questions or concerns about your medication. No medication plan is etched in stone. You'll get the best results when you understand your plan and agree to follow it.

Simple analgesics

Analgesics (an-ul-JE-ziks) are medications specifically designed to reduce or relieve pain. They control pain in various ways by interfering with the ways in which pain messages are developed, transmitted or interpreted. Simple analgesics are different from opioid medications — also known as narcotics — described later in this chapter.

The following are common OTC and prescription pain relievers.

Nonsteroidal anti-inflammatory drugs (NSAIDs)

NSAIDs (en-SEDS) are most effective for mild to moderate pain accompanied by swelling and inflammation. These drugs relieve pain by inhibiting an enzyme in your body called cyclooxygenase (si-klo-OX-suh-juhn-ays). This enzyme makes hormone-like substances called prostaglandins, which are involved in the development of pain and inflammation.

NSAIDs are especially helpful for arthritis and pain resulting from muscle sprains, strains, back and neck injuries or cramps.

Over-the-counter NSAIDs include:

- Aspirin
- Ibuprofen (Advil, Motrin, others)
- Ketoprofen (Orudis)
- Naproxen sodium (Aleve)

NSAIDs available only by prescription include:

- Diclofenac potassium (Cataflam)
- Diclofenac sodium (Voltaren)
- Etodolac (Lodine)
- Fenoprofen (Nalfon)
- Flurbiprofen (Ansaid)
- Indomethacin (Indocin)
- Ketorolac (Toradol)
- Nabumetone (Relafen)
- Naproxen (Anaprox DS, Naprelan, Naprosyn)
- Oxaprozin (Daypro)
- Piroxicam (Feldene)
- Sulindac (Clinoril)

When taken as directed, NSAIDs are generally safe. But if you take more than the recommended dosage — and sometimes even the recommended dosage — NSAIDs may cause nausea, stomach pain, stomach bleeding or ulcers. Large doses of NSAIDs can also lead to kidney problems and fluid retention. Risk of these conditions increases with age. If you regularly take NSAIDs, talk to your doctor so that he or she can monitor for side effects.

NSAIDs also have a so-called ceiling effect, or limit to how much pain they can control. This means that beyond a certain dosage, they don't provide additional benefit. If you have moderate to severe pain, exceeding the dosage limit may not help to relieve your pain.

COX-2 inhibitors

Newer NSAIDs include these prescription drugs:

- Celecoxib (Celebrex)
- Valdecoxib (Bextra)

Cyclooxygenase comes in two forms, called COX-1 and COX-2. Unlike other NSAIDs, COX-2 inhibitors suppress only one form of cyclooxygenase. Researchers believe part of the role of COX-1 is to protect your stomach lining. Because NSAIDs suppress its function, side effects such as stomach and bleeding problems can result.

COX-2 inhibitors affect only that form of the enzyme (COX-2) involved in inflammation. Because they don't affect COX-1, COX-2 inhibitors may cause fewer side effects in your digestive system. However, this result, along with the long-term effects of COX-2 inhibitors, needs to be verified with further research. In addition, COX-2 inhibitors don't thin the blood like aspirin and other NSAIDs. If your doctor has prescribed aspirin for a heart condition, COX-2 inhibitors aren't a substitute.

Acetaminophen

Acetaminophen (Tylenol, others) is most effective for mild to moderate pain that isn't accompanied by inflammation. Unlike COX-2 inhibitors and other NSAIDs, acetaminophen doesn't affect prostaglandins. Therefore, it does little to reduce inflammation.

When taken occasionally and as recommended, acetaminophen is safe. However, if you frequently take more of the drug than recommended on the product label, you risk liver or kidney damage. Taking acetaminophen with alcohol increases that risk and can lead to sudden and severe problems such as liver failure. If you frequently take acetaminophen, tell your doctor so that he or she can monitor side effects.

Acetaminophen and NSAIDS are sometimes combined with an opioid to provide stronger pain relief. These drugs are available only by prescription. Whenever you use a combination of medications, ask your doctor and pharmacist about the use and side effects of each individual drug.

Opioids (narcotics)

Opioids are prescription medications and are regulated as controlled substances by the Drug Enforcement Administration. A doctor must have a special license in order to prescribe these drugs.

Opioids are often used to relieve pain from cancer, terminal illness, severe injury or surgery. Pain control after surgery is especially important. The sooner you're active, the less the risk of complications due to inactivity, such as pneumonia or blood clots.

Opioids, sometimes called narcotics, come in several forms. Some are natural compounds derived from the opium poppy. These compounds are called opiates. There are also synthetic opioids that work in similar ways. *Opioids* include both these natural and synthetic forms and is the preferred term.

Your body contains naturally occurring chemicals called opioid peptides that are similar to morphine. One theory behind several complementary and alternative treatments for pain (see Chapter 7) is that they activate naturally occurring opioid peptides in your brain and spinal cord.

Commonly used opioids
Frequently prescribed opioids include the following:
- Codeine
- Fentanyl (Duragesic)
- Hydrocodone
- Hydromorphone (Dilaudid)
- Levorphanol (Levo-Dromoran)
- Meperidine (Demerol)
- Methadone (Dolophine)
- Morphine (MS Contin, Oramorph SR, others)
- Oxycodone (OxyContin)
- Oxymorphone (Numorphan)
- Propoxyphene (Darvon)

Side effects of opioids can include mild dizziness, drowsiness, sedation and unclear thinking. These can make it unsafe for you to drive or operate machinery. Sometimes you can do things to manage dizziness. For example, you might feel better after lying down for a while. Getting up slowly from a sitting or lying position also can help. If you experience severe dizziness or drowsiness, get emergency care. Also go to the emergency room if you feel extreme nervousness, severe weakness, cold, clammy skin or have trouble breathing.

Other side effects of opioids include constipation, nausea and vomiting. Ask your doctor or pharmacist about ways to manage these.

Tramadol

Tramadol (Ultram) is a prescription pain medication that works in two ways. Like an opioid, it interferes with the transmission of pain signals. The drug also triggers release of norepinephrine (nor-ep-i-NEF-rin) and serotonin — neurotransmitters that help reduce pain.

Tramadol is used mainly to relieve moderate to severe acute pain. Its effect in treating chronic pain hasn't been well studied. In a few studies where the drug was prescribed for chronic pain, some people experienced significant pain relief and others got no relief at all.

Because it's not a true opioid, risk of physical dependence and addiction is less. Side effects from tramadol can include dizziness, sedation, headache, nausea, constipation and seizures. Possible long-term effects from the drug are unknown.

The medical debate over opioids

The goal of treatment of acute pain is to relieve pain immediately, usually with medications. Unrelieved pain has many negative effects, such as delayed recovery from surgery and decreased immunity to disease.

For people with chronic pain, the goals of treatment are more complex. Pain relief is important, but so is the ability to function at work and to be able to enjoy social and leisure activities.

The goal of pain relief and the goal of improved function are sometimes in conflict. Opioids are powerful pain relievers. When taken in small amounts for short periods, opioids generally cause only minor side effects. But when opioids are taken in increasing doses for several weeks or months, these side effects can become bothersome.

Opioids can also have an effect sometimes described as rebound pain. For instance, some opioids have an effect that lasts only a few hours. Pain can recur as these short-acting medications wear off or when they are withdrawn from your treatment plan.

Ironically, opioids can also cause changes in your nervous system that actually may heighten your perception of pain and make you feel more uncomfortable. This condition is called hyperalgesia.

In summary, opioids have many effects, some good and some bad. For this reason, plus concerns about lack of effectiveness for some types of pain, some doctors restrict the use of opioids when treating chronic pain. They may also be uneasy about possible long-term side effects of opioids, which can interfere with rehabilitation and lead to more doctor visits and hospital stays. They also cite the risk of physical dependence and addiction to opioids.

Other doctors take the position that withholding opioids leads to unnecessary pain and suffering, that side effects of opioids can be managed and that the risk of addiction is overblown. This view holds that legal and medically supervised use of opioids has little in common with illegal use of such drugs.

Getting clear about the risk of addiction
The issue of addiction is important. Many discussions about it get confused because people use three terms synonymously: *tolerance*, *physical dependence* and *addiction*. In fact, these words point to three different conditions:

- **Tolerance** happens when the initial dose of an opioid loses its effectiveness over time, calling for higher doses of the drug to produce the desired effect.
- **Physical dependence** occurs when your body adapts to a drug. When the drug is withdrawn, you may then experience anxiety, tremors and other physical withdrawal symptoms.
- **Addiction** is a primary disease marked by cravings for a drug and compulsive use of that drug despite repeated, harmful consequences.

With time, people who take opioids are likely to develop tolerance and even physical dependence. However, this doesn't mean that they are addicted to opioids. Addiction results from many factors — genetic, psychological and environmental — and often takes years to develop. Exposure to opioids is only one factor. Most people treated with opioids never become addicted.

Sometimes, people with chronic pain act in ways that are mistakenly called addictive. These people may focus on maintaining their supply of opioids or closely watch the clock to make sure they take their next dose of medication. Often these are not addictive behaviors but pseudoaddiction — behaviors that stop once people get satisfactory pain relief.

Considering opioids in your pain treatment

Despite the debate over the use of opioids, they can be a key part of your treatment plan. Before prescribing these drugs, your doctor will give you a thorough physical exam and take a detailed medical history. The results will help determine whether opioids are right for you.

When thinking about opioids, consider your full range of options. Ask about the possibility of combining opioids with simple analgesics for maximum pain relief.

Compare the benefits of short-acting and sustained-release medications, and discuss whether you should take opioids on a regular schedule or simply on an as-needed basis. In addition, before taking opioids, you may want to get a second opinion.

Finally, after you start taking an opioid, compare your function and activity levels with how you were functioning before you began taking the medication. You'll want to see a marked improvement before deciding to continue using the medication long term.

Topical medications

Topical medications are creams or gels that are applied to the skin. These drugs act on the surface of your body or are absorbed through the skin. Pain relief ointments can occasionally help relieve nerve pain and inflammation just below the surface of your skin. Three types of topical medications are available. They are local anesthetics, analgesics and counter-irritant products.

Local anesthetics

EMLA. EMLA is a prescription pain relief cream made from two topical anesthetics — lidocaine and prilocaine. Your skin becomes numb within an hour after application, and the benefits are greatest 2 to 3 hours following application. EMLA is commonly used — especially on children — to reduce pain before giving a shot, drawing blood, inserting an intravenous line or treating a wart.

Lidocaine patch. A lidocaine patch (Lidoderm) may be prescribed for relief of pain associated with postherpetic neuralgia and nerve pain.

Over-the-counter products. There are several OTC topical medications available for pain relief. They include dibucaine (Nupercainal), lidocaine (Xylocaine, Zilactin-L), benzocaine (Lanacane, Solarcain) and pramoxine (Prax, Itch-X).

Analgesics

Capsaicin. This nonprescription drug is made from the seeds of hot chili peppers. It's thought to work by depleting nerve cells of a chemical called substance P, which has a role in transmitting pain messages.

You rub capsaicin (Capzasin-P, Dolorac, Zostrix) on your skin, typically three or five times a day. It usually takes up to 1 to 2 weeks before you begin to feel noticeable pain relief. If you miss one or two applications, it will take longer for the drug to work.

Capsaicin is most effective for temporary relief of arthritic pain in joints close to your skin's surface, such as your fingers, knees and elbows. It may also help relieve pain after shingles (postherpetic neuralgia), pain from diabetes (diabetic neuropathy) and chronic pain near healed surgical scars.

Because the drug is generally safe and effective, you can use it long term. However, because it can temporarily irritate your skin and produce a burning sensation, wear rubber gloves when applying capsaicin and be careful not to get it in your eyes.

Trolamine salicylate. Medications such as Aspercreme, Sportscreme and Myoflex contain trolamine salicylate (TRO-luh-mene suh-LIS-uh-late), a chemical that's similar to aspirin. The Food and Drug Administration (FDA) lists these drugs as safe, but not necessarily effective for pain relief. They are available over-the-counter.

Counter-irritant products

These nonprescription medications (ArthriCare, Ben-Gay, Icy Hot) stimulate your sensory receptors of heat or cold to cover up or counter pain.

Counter-irritant products may relieve occasional, mild muscle aches, but they're not effective for most forms of chronic pain. In addition, they typically require frequent applications, and some products have a medicinal smell.

Other medications for pain treatment

Some of the more effective and commonly used medications for chronic pain are drugs that were developed to control other conditions, such as depression and seizures. The following auxiliary, or adjuvant medications typically don't fall under the heading of analgesics but can also reduce pain.

Tricyclic antidepressants

In addition to relieving symptoms of depression, these drugs interfere with certain chemical processes in your brain that cause you to feel pain.

They include:

- Amitriptyline (Elavil)
- Desipramine (Norpramin)
- Doxepin (Sinequan)
- Imipramine (Tofranil)
- Nortriptyline (Aventyl, Pamelor)
- Protriptyline (Vivactil)

Antidepressants don't cause dependence or addiction. However, tricyclic antidepressants can make you drowsy. Therefore, it's generally recommended that you take the medication in the evening before bed. In addition, these drugs may cause dry mouth, constipation, difficulty with urination, weight gain and changes in blood pressure. Side effects usually begin soon after you start taking the medication or your dose is increased, but the pain relief may not occur for several weeks.

To reduce or prevent these symptoms, your doctor will likely start you off at a low dose and slowly increase the amount. Most people are able to take tricyclic antidepressants, particularly in low doses, with only mild side effects.

Antiseizure medications
Developed primarily to reduce or control epileptic seizures, these medications also help control stabbing or shooting pain from nerve damage. These drugs seem to work by quieting damaged nerves to slow or prevent uncontrolled pain signals.

Antiseizure medications used for chronic pain include:
- Carbamazepine (Carbatrol, Tegretol)
- Clonazepam (Klonopin)
- Divalproex sodium (Depakote)
- Gabapentin (Neurontin)
- Lamotrigine (Lamictal)
- Phenytoin (Dilantin)
- Oxcarbazepine (Trileptal)
- Tiagabine (Gabitril)
- Topiramate (Topamax)
- Valproic acid (Depakene)

These medications can cause dizziness, drowsiness, nausea and lack of balance and coordination. But, again, most people are bothered only minimally. More severe but less common side effects include blood and liver disorders. To reduce your risk of side effects, your doctor will likely start you off on a small amount of the drug and gradually increase the dose while monitoring you.

Medications for associated symptoms

Relief from your pain isn't the only reason you may take medication. Drugs may not reduce your pain, but they can relieve other troubling symptoms associated with chronic pain. This is important because when you aren't affected by other symptoms, you can direct more of your energy toward your daily activities.

Depression

Depression is common among people who have chronic pain. Relief from depression can have a significant effect on your ability to manage your pain. As you begin to feel better and more energetic, your pain seems more tolerable.

Experts believe depression may result from an imbalance in certain brain chemicals (neurotransmitters) that affect your mood and emotions. The condition is often treated with medications that increase production of these chemicals. In addition to tricyclic antidepressants discussed earlier, other types of antidepressants include:

Selective serotonin reuptake inhibitors (SSRIs). These medications have become a first-line treatment for depression because they produce few serious side effects. The drugs seem to work by increasing the availability of the neurotransmitter serotonin.

SSRIs include the prescription medications:

- Citalopram (Celexa)
- Fluoxetine (Prozac, Sarafem)
- Fluvoxamine (Luvox)
- Paroxetine (Paxil)
- Sertraline (Zoloft)

SSRIs can cause sexual problems in up to 30 percent of people. However, once you stop taking the drug, the problems usually go away.

Other antidepressants work in ways similar to SSRIs but may affect different neurotransmitters. These include:

- Bupropion (Wellbutrin)
- Maprotiline
- Mirtazapine (Remeron)
- Nefazodone (Serzone)
- Trazodone (Desyrel)
- Venlafaxine (Effexor)

Monoamine oxidase inhibitors. These drugs are generally prescribed only if other antidepressants aren't effective. They include:

- Isocarboxazid (Marplan)
- Phenelzine (Nardil)
- Tranylcypromine (Parnate)

These drugs can interact with certain foods and other medications to cause serious side effects, including chest pain, labored breathing and an increase in your blood pressure and heart rate. Less serious and more common side effects include feeling light-headed or dizzy.

Mood-stabilizing medications. This group of drugs is used to treat bipolar disorder (manic-depressive illness), which involves extreme, recurrent cycles of elation and depression.

These medications include:

- Carbamazepine (Carbatrol, Tegretol)
- Divalproex sodium (Depakote)
- Gabapentin (Neurontin)
- Lithium (Eskalith, Lithobid)
- Valproic acid (Depakene)

Insomnia

A good night's sleep can help you better cope with your pain by renewing your energy level and improving your mood. Medications that promote sleep include:

Antidepressants. Drowsiness is a common side effect of some antidepressants. When taken at night before bed, the drugs may help you sleep better — in addition to controlling pain and depression.

Sedatives. These medications help promote sleep. However, they can cloud your thinking, make you drowsy, impair your balance and affect your ability to drive, especially when taken in combination with opioids. If taken regularly, they may also cause dependency or addiction.

Prescription sedatives include:

- Alprazolam (Xanax)
- Butabarbital sodium (Butisol Sodium)
- Chlordiazepoxide (Librium)
- Clonazepam (Klonopin)
- Clorazepate (Tranxene)
- Diazepam (Valium)
- Estazolam (ProSom)

- Flurazepam (Dalmane)
- Lorazepam (Ativan)
- Oxazepam (Serax)
- Pentobarbital (Nembutal)
- Quazepam (Doral)
- Temazepam (Restoril)
- Triazolam (Halcion)
- Zaleplon (Sonata)
- Zolpidem (Ambien)

Zaleplon and zolpidem are newer types of sleep medication that promote more natural sleep. These drugs aren't as likely to lead to dependence as other sedatives.

Muscle spasms

If your pain is accompanied by muscle spasms, your doctor may recommend a muscle relaxant to control the spasms. Various side effects are possible. For example, these drugs can cloud your thinking and leave you drowsy and dizzy, especially when taken in combination with opioids.

Muscle relaxants include these prescription drugs:
- Baclofen (Lioresal)
- Carisoprodol (Soma)
- Chlorzoxazone (Parafon Forte)
- Cyclobenzaprine (Flexeril)
- Methocarbamol (Robaxin)
- Orphenadrine (Norflex)
- Tizanidine (Zanaflex)

Inflammation

If your pain is associated with rheumatoid arthritis, your doctor may prescribe an anti-inflammatory drug, including NSAIDs and steroids. Such treatment is designed both to ease the pain and to reduce the inflammation that may damage your joints.

If you have an acutely inflamed joint, NSAIDs may not be effective and your doctor may prescribe a corticosteroid. Corticosteroids may be given for short-term or long-term treatment.

Some of the leading corticosteroids include:
- Cortisone
- Methylprednisolone (Medrol)
- Prednisolone
- Triamcinolone (Aristocort)

Medications for specific pain conditions

Your doctor might prescribe medications for specific pain conditions. Examples of these conditions include migraines and irritable bowel syndrome.

Medications for migraines
If your migraines don't respond to common pain medications, your doctor may recommend drugs specifically for this condition.

Medications to prevent or reduce the frequency of migraines include:
- **Cardiovascular drugs.** These include beta blockers and calcium channel blockers. How they control migraines is unclear.
- **Antidepressants.** Tricyclic antidepressants increase levels of some neurotransmitters in the brain.
- **Antiseizure drugs.** Valproic acid (Depakene) is an example. Its mechanism of action on migraines is uncertain.
- **Serotonin antagonists.** Drugs such as cyproheptadine (Periactin) and methylsergide (Sansert) affect levels of serotonin.
- **Riboflavin (vitamin B 2).** A riboflavin deficiency may contribute to recurring headaches. High doses of vitamin B 2 (400 milligrams a day) may correct the deficiency. Take high doses of this vitamin only with medical supervision.
- **Botulinum toxin type A (Botox).** This drug has been approved by the FDA for temporarily improving the appearance of moderate-to-severe frown lines between the eyebrows (glabellar lines). In clinical studies, specially targeted injections of botulinum toxin type A have reduced both the frequency and intensity of migraines in some people.

Other drugs that help relieve symptoms after a migraine starts include:

- **Triptans.** These drugs mimic the brain chemical serotonin, deactivating nerves and shrinking swollen blood vessels. Sumatriptan (Imitrex) comes in pill, injection and nasal spray form. Similar drugs include naratriptan (Amerge), rizatriptan (Maxalt), zolmitriptan (Zomig) and almotriptan (Axert).
- **Ergotamines.** The drugs dihydroergotamine (Migranal, D.H.E. 45) and ergotamine (Ergomar) influence brain hormone receptors, including serotonin receptors.
- **Mixed analgesics.** They include Fioricet, Fiorinal and Midrin, which contain a combination of medications, including acetaminophen.
- **Lidocaine nasal drops.** They contain an anesthetic that works on nasal passage nerves. The drops often relieve pain within a few minutes, but in about 40 percent of people the pain returns.

Medications for irritable bowel syndrome

Irritable bowel syndrome (IBS) is characterized by abdominal pain or cramping and changes in bowel function. These changes can include bloating, gas, diarrhea and constipation.

An estimated 35 million Americans have irritable bowel syndrome. It ranks second only to the common cold as a cause of lost work time and accounts for about 3 million doctor visits in the United States every year. Because it's still not clear what causes IBS, treatment focuses on the relief of symptoms so that you can live your life as fully and normally as possible.

In most cases, you can successfully control mild symptoms of IBS by learning to manage stress and making changes in your diet and lifestyle. But if your symptoms are moderate or severe, you may need more help than lifestyle changes alone can offer.

For moderate symptoms of IBS, your doctor may suggest:

- **Fiber supplements.** These include psyllium and methylcellulose.
- **Over-the-counter medications.** Drugs such as loperamide (Imodium) can help control diarrhea. Constipation may be helped by docusate (Colace) or extract of senna (Senokot).

- **Anticholinergics.** These drugs affect certain activities of the nervous system to relieve painful bowel spasms. They include dicyclomine (Bentyl) and hyoscyamine (Levsin).
- **Antidepressants.** Besides relieving depression, these medications can slow the activity of neurons that control your intestinal function. For diarrhea and abdominal pain, your doctor may suggest tricyclic antidepressants such as imipramine (Tofranil) and amitriptyline (Elavil). Side effects of these drugs include drowsiness, dry mouth and constipation. Selective serotonin reuptake inhibitors such as fluoxetine (Prozac, Sarafem), paroxetine (Paxil) and others may help if you're depressed and have pain and constipation. Sometimes, SSRIs don't help, and in such cases, counseling may achieve some positive results.

If you have severe IBS, it's important to receive ongoing treatment and support from your doctor.

In November 2000, the FDA approved the first medication specifically for the treatment of moderate to severe IBS in women. Alosetron (Lotronex) is a nerve receptor antagonist that's designed to relax the colon and slow the movement of waste through the lower bowel. Due to safety concerns, Lotronex was pulled from the market in late November 2000 at the urging of the FDA. It's now available but with strict guidelines for use. Be sure to discuss these with your doctor.

Chapter 6

Technologies for treating pain

Medical technology offers several choices for treating chronic pain. Options range from using needles to inject medication at or near the site of your pain to implanting complex devices, including nerve stimulators and medication pumps, in your body.

Injections

Instead of prescribing pills to control pain, your doctor might inject medication. Injections typically don't cure pain, but they may help you through an initial period of intense pain or a flare-up of severe pain.

Injections are most effective for joint, muscle or nerve pain that's confined to a specific location. Injected medications may be an anesthetic to control the pain, a steroid to reduce inflammation or a combination of the two. In addition, a substance that improves joint mobility is also sometimes used.

One benefit of injections is that the medication works primarily in a limited part of your body. By targeting a specific area, injections may reduce the amount of medication needed and the number and intensity of side effects.

Injections can also help in diagnosing the cause of your pain. Suppose, for example, that a small amount of anesthetic injected at a specific location relieves your pain. This may indicate that the pain is coming primarily from that joint, muscle or nerve.

In deciding whether injections may be right for you, keep in mind that you'll have to visit your doctor's office for each shot. In addition, the site of the injection and the type of medication used can limit how often you receive an injection. For instance, injected steroids may cause adverse side effects that become worse with frequent use.

Injections are seldom used by themselves to treat chronic pain. Rather, they're usually used in conjunction with a program that includes physical therapy. Injections can make such therapy more comfortable.

The types of injections can be divided into three broad categories: joint injections, soft tissue injections and nerve block injections.

Joint injections

When joints become inflamed and painful, your doctor may inject medications into them to ease your discomfort. Two types of medications are used for joint injections. They are corticosteroids and hyaluronic acid.

Corticosteroids. If arthritis has caused your joints to become inflamed, swollen and painful, your physician may suggest injecting the affected joint with a corticosteroid.

Corticosteroids mimic the effects of the hormones cortisone and hydrocortisone, which are made by the outer layer (cortex) of your adrenal glands. When prescribed in doses that exceed your natural-occurring levels, corticosteroids suppress inflammation. They are injected into one or several affected areas of your body, such as the shoulder, elbow, hip or knee. Some joint injections, such as facet or sacroiliac injections, are given in the spine.

In the short term, corticosteroids can make you feel dramatically better. But when used for many months or years, they may become less effective and cause serious side effects. Side effects can include weakened cartilage and ligaments, easy bruising, thinning of bones, cataracts, weight gain, a round face, diabetes and high blood pressure.

Corticosteroid injections may offer some pain relief for 4 to 6 months.

Hyaluronic acid. Hyaluronate (Hyalgan) and hylan G-F 20 (Synvisc) are injectable drugs that are used to treat osteoarthritis of the knee.

Hyaluronic acid is a substance found in normal joint fluid. Joint fluid acts as a lubricant. Hyaluronate and hylan G-F 20 help relieve pain by supplementing hyaluronic acid in the joint. These drugs may be offered to people who can't get relief from exercise, physical therapy or other pain medication. Because they're injected directly into the knee, hyaluronate and hylan G-F 20 don't cause the side effects of oral pain medications.

Hyaluronate is administered in a series of five injections — one per week — into the knee joint. A local anesthetic is injected first to ease discomfort from the hyaluronate, which is thick and must be administered with a large-gauge needle. Relief may last up to 12 months.

Hylan G-F 20 is given in three injections. Relief may last 6 months or longer. Both drugs usually bring pain relief more slowly than do corticosteroids. Hylan G-F 20 shouldn't be given to people who are allergic to eggs.

The effectiveness of hyaluronate injections for treating chronic knee pain associated with osteoarthritis is still being studied.

Soft tissue injections

When specific parts of your body — such as a muscle or bursa — are inflamed and painful, injections can be given directly into the surrounding soft tissue.

Trigger point or field block injections. Trigger points are areas where your muscles and surrounding fibrous (fascial) tissue are sensitive to touch. Trigger points are generally in the upper and lower back muscles, but they may occur elsewhere. Trigger point injections are used when muscles are sensitive to touch and are the source of pain. Depending on the medication used, trigger point injections can reduce pain in the muscle, reduce inflammation or relax a muscle.

Your doctor may inject your muscle with a preparation of local anesthetic and corticosteroid. This may reduce pain and promote increased movement. The local anesthetic initially numbs the area to reduce pain while the corticosteroid reduces inflammation. The corticosteroid begins working in 3 to 4 days and may provide long-term reduction of inflammation and pain. Sometimes an anesthetic alone is used if there is little or no inflammation and the goal is to relax the muscle for more effective stretching.

Bursa injections. Bursa are tiny, fluid-filled sacs that lubricate and cushion pressure points between your bones and the tendons and muscles near your joints. You have more than 150 bursae in your body, and they help you move without pain. When bursae become inflamed (bursitis), movement of or pressure on the affected joint is painful.

Bursitis most often affects the shoulder, elbow or hip areas. Injections of corticosteroid can be given to reduce inflammation.

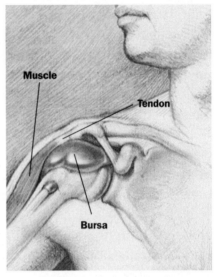

Corticosteroid injections are sometimes given to reduce pain associated with bursitis. Medication is injected directly into the affected area.

Nerve block injections

To do a nerve block, your doctor will inject an anesthetic around a nerve's fibers. This prevents pain messages that are traveling along that nerve pathway from reaching your brain.

Nerve blocks are most often used to relieve pain for a short period, such as during surgery. If there is inflammation around a nerve, an injection of corticosteroid in conjunction with the nerve block may provide longer pain relief.

There are three main types of nerve blocks:

Peripheral. For localized pain, an anesthetic is injected around a nerve that's away from the spine, such as in an ankle. The result is reduced feeling and less pain in that area.

Spinal. For pain that affects a broader area, such as your lower back or a leg, an anesthetic is injected in or near the spinal column. An injection directly into the spinal fluid is called an intrathecal (in-truh-THEE-kul) injection. This type of injection is often used during surgery on the abdomen or lower extremities.

If the injection isn't into the spinal fluid, it's called an epidural (ep-ih-DUR-ul) injection. Epidurals are often used to relieve the pain of childbirth and sometimes to relieve some types of back pain, such as sciatica.

Sympathetic. Some forms of chronic pain, such as complex regional pain syndrome (CRPS), formerly called reflex sympathetic dystrophy (RSD), may result from abnormal activity of your sympathetic nervous system. Your sympathetic nerves control circulation and perspiration and are part of your autonomic nervous system. Injection of an anesthetic to block the sympathetic nerves may relieve pain.

Nerve stimulators and medication pumps

Nerve stimulators include transcutaneous electronic nerve stimulators (TENS), spinal cord stimulators and peripheral nerve stimulators.

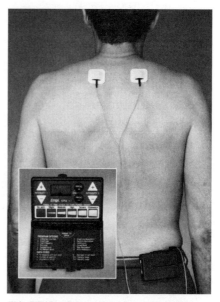

TENS
For this type of nerve stimulation, electrodes are placed on your skin near the painful area. The electrodes are then attached to a small, portable, battery-powered unit. The unit generates low-level, painless electric impulses that pass through your skin to nearby nerve pathways in your body. You adjust settings on the TENS unit as needed to control pain.

This TENS unit has electrodes placed for the treatment of neck pain. The lightweight unit is carried in your pocket, purse or on your belt. A control panel in the unit allows you to select the level of electric impulse.

Exactly how TENS works isn't known. It may trigger the release of endorphins — chemicals in your body that have painkilling effects similar to morphine. TENS treatment may also block nerve pathways that carry pain messages.

TENS generally works best for acute pain from a pinched nerve. This technology may be less successful for treating chronic pain, although some people with chronic pain do benefit from it. Most often, TENS is used along with exercise and other pain treatments.

A similar and newer treatment called percutaneous electronic nerve stimulation (PENS) is now under study. Like TENS, this technology delivers an electric current to your nerves. But instead of transmitting the current through electrodes placed on top of your skin, PENS uses needles that penetrate your skin to just below the surface. These needles are quite thin, like those used in acupuncture. Most people feel some sensation, but not pain, when these needles are inserted.

Spinal cord and peripheral nerve stimulators

Using technologies more complicated than TENS, spinal cord and peripheral nerve stimulators act directly on large nerve bundles involved in pain transmission. How they moderate pain isn't completely understood, but it's thought they may affect production of specific chemicals in your nervous system called neurotransmitters.

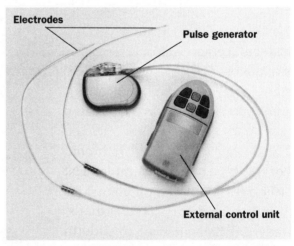

The spinal cord stimulator pulse generator is implanted below the skin in your abdomen or upper part of your buttocks with electrodes attached near your spinal cord. A handheld touch-pad control unit allows you to control the level of stimulation.

Spinal cord and peripheral nerve stimulators use the same kind of technology as pacemakers, which generate electric currents to stimulate a heartbeat. The current from nerve stimulators produces subtle, tingling sensations that can block or mask the feeling of pain. Like pacemakers, nerve stimulators can be implanted in your body.

Medication pumps

Medication pumps, also called pain pumps or morphine pumps, can be used for a wide range of problems. These include chronic pain as well as pain from nerve damage or illness.

Most often a medication pump is surgically placed in the lower abdomen. The pump is programmable and provides an adjustable flow of medication to the spinal column. Typically the medication is an opioid, which may be combined with a local anesthetic.

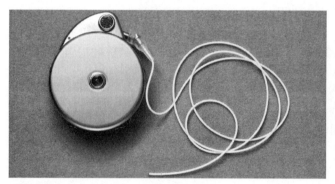

The implantable medication pump supplies pain medication directly to the spinal fluid through a small tube. The pump is replenished by injecting drugs through the skin and into the small port at the center of the unit.

Choosing a technology that works for you

The technologies described in this chapter offer a variety of treatment options. Keep in mind that these options don't exclude one another. For instance, someone with chronic pain could use an implanted medication pump along with a TENS unit in conjunction with a physical therapy program.

Choosing the technology that's best for you at any given time is a decision that involves considering several factors. Be sure to discuss the issues below — as well as any other questions you have — with your doctor.

Your expectations. Stimulators and medication pumps represent the latest in pain management technology. However, no technology offers total pain relief. Technology can lessen your discomfort, but you'll probably continue to feel some pain. A reasonable goal is to reduce your pain by 50 percent.

A related factor is the overall goal of treatment. Some people with chronic pain expect to lead active lives — to return to work and to normal family life. Rehabilitation is their primary aim. Over the long term, these people can supplement technology with other methods for treating pain.

For people in the last stages of an incurable cancer or another end-stage illness, immediate relief of pain may be the most important goal.

Your treatment history. Before prescribing devices such as implantable stimulators and pumps, your doctor may first try a variety of other treatments, such as oral medication, physical therapy, counseling and exercise.

Your doctor will probably recommend a "high-tech" treatment only after you've tried less invasive and less expensive options. Knowing how you've responded to pain treatments in the past can help predict how well a new technology may work for you.

Your medical evaluation. Before trying a stimulator or pump, you'll undergo a physical exam and medical history. Your doctor might also order tests such as a magnetic resonance imaging (MRI) or a computerized tomography (CT) scan.

Your doctor will probably also require that you have a psychological evaluation. This step isn't meant to imply that you're mentally ill or that the pain is just in your head. Instead, psychological evaluation recognizes that your mind and body are connected. The success of any medical treatment may depend in part on your feelings about it as well as the day-to-day behaviors that you use to cope with pain.

Conditions such as depression and anxiety may exist along with chronic pain. These conditions can affect your experience of pain and how you respond to it. So in addition to technology, your doctor might recommend counseling as a way to help you make lasting changes in your attitude and behavior.

Medical risks and side effects. Surgery is needed to implant any device in your body, and any surgery carries some risk. In addition, pain medications have side effects — a factor to consider with injections or any device that delivers medication. In addition, there's an ongoing risk of infection with an implanted device.

One advantage of pain pumps is that they deliver medication directly to your spinal column. This allows your doctor to prescribe lower doses than with oral drugs. In turn, the lower doses can reduce side effects.

Your range of pain. When chronic pain seems localized in a particular area of your body, peripheral nerve stimulation may be the best option. For pain that spreads over a larger region of your body, spinal cord stimulators or medication pumps might be more useful. But again, no technology offers total pain relief.

Your comfort level. Some pumps and stimulators come with handheld programmers, which you'll have to learn to use. In addition, these devices are battery-powered. From time to time the battery packs must be changed. Pumps also must be refilled with medication.

Like any piece of technology, pumps and stimulators require general maintenance and troubleshooting. Sometimes the entire device needs to be replaced, requiring another round of surgery.

Be sure that you fully understand all of the instructions for using a pump or stimulator. You'll want to avoid situations that cause your device to malfunction. For example, you can't have an MRI while using a spinal cord stimulator.

It's important to understand the limitations of these devices as you consider their use over less complicated therapies.

You and your doctor. Using any technology may mean more frequent visits to your doctor's office. You'll see each other regularly to monitor your device, assess results of the therapy and keep your stimulator or pump well maintained. You'll need to communicate openly with your doctor and work as a team.

Where you live and travel. If your stimulator malfunctions or your pump runs out of medication, you may experience withdrawal symptoms, changes in blood pressure or other complications. During such a situation, you'll need to get to a doctor. This may be a factor in choosing where to live and work. It may also be a factor to consider when making travel plans.

Insurance coverage. Although pain-relief technologies are expensive, most medical insurers will cover the cost of their implantation and use. You'll need to work with your doctor and insurance company in order to satisfy requirements for coverage.

Trial run. Before committing to use a medical device over the long term, you'll typically use it for a brief trial period to see if it helps. Health insurers often require this trial run before they cover the cost of implanting a device.

To do a trial, you'll use an external stimulator or pump in a hospital or outpatient setting. After the test period, you'll know much more about how well you'll tolerate the device and how much pain relief it can deliver. In addition, trying it out before implantation allows you to avoid surgery if the technology doesn't work for you.

Chapter 7

Complementary and alternative medicine

I n your effort to find relief from pain, chances are you've tried or considered some form of complementary or alternative medicine. Maybe you've had a massage, practiced meditation or yoga or thought about acupuncture or herbal medicines.

And you probably have a lot of questions. Do these methods really work? Are they safe? Exactly what is complementary and alternative medicine? This chapter offers answers to these questions.

Defining complementary and alternative medicine

The National Center for Complementary and Alternative Medicine (NCCAM), a division of the National Institutes of Health (NIH), defines complementary and alternative medicine as treatments and health care practices that aren't widely taught in medical schools, not generally used in hospitals and not usually reimbursed by health insurance companies. Examples might be practicing tai chi — in addition to taking medication prescribed by your doctor — to treat back pain or using an herbal preparation instead of traditional chemotherapy or radiation to treat cancer.

Often, the emphasis of complementary and alternative medicine is on a holistic approach that considers physical, mental, emotional and spiritual aspects of health. Preventing health problems rather than treating them also is stressed. Some complementary and alternative therapies are consistent with conventional medicine while others aren't accepted in conventional practice.

Options available

Complementary and alternative therapies aren't new. Some have been practiced for thousands of years. But their use has become more popular as people seek greater control of their own health. Two of the most common problems for which people use complementary and alternative medicine are anxiety and pain. Studies conducted under the auspices of NCCAM have shown that biofeedback, meditation and relaxation techniques can be useful in treating insomnia and chronic pain.

Following are brief summaries of common complementary and alternative treatments that have been promoted for pain management. Before you try any of them, be sure to read "Five steps in considering any treatment" at the end of this chapter.

Acupressure

Acupressure, like acupuncture, stems from the Chinese belief that just below your skin are 14 invisible pathways, called meridians. Through these pathways flows chi (chee), the Chinese word for "life force." When the flow of chi is interrupted, illness results.

During acupressure, a practitioner applies pressure with his or her fingers to specific points on your body to restore free flow of chi and relieve symptoms such as pain and stress.

Many people who feel they're helped by the procedure find this hands-on therapy to be relaxing and comforting. Research is still needed to document the effectiveness of this treatment.

Acupuncture

During a typical acupuncture session, an acupuncturist inserts anywhere from 1 to 20 hair-thin needles into your skin for 10 to 30 minutes. The purpose of the needles is to remove blockages in the meridians and promote the free flow of chi. The acupuncturist may also manipulate the needles or apply electrical stimulation or heat to the needles. There should be little or no pain from insertion of the needles.

Acupuncture is one of the most studied unconventional medical practices, and it's gaining acceptance into Westernized medicine for treatment of certain conditions. A 1997 consensus statement released by the NIH stated there is clear evidence that acupuncture helps relieve postoperative dental pain and that it's also useful in treating nausea following surgery and chemotherapy. In addition, acupuncture can play a useful role in treatment for addiction, stroke rehabilitation, headache, menstrual cramps, tennis elbow, myofascial pain, osteoarthritis, low back pain, carpal tunnel syndrome and asthma. It's most useful when used as part of a multidisciplinary approach to treating these conditions.

Adverse side effects from acupuncture are rare, but they can occur. Make sure your acupuncturist is trained and follows good hygiene practices, including use of disposable needles.

Aromatherapy

This ancient form of healing uses essential oils derived from plant extracts and resins to promote both health and beauty. Practitioners believe these oils can help treat various conditions — including chronic pain — when massaged into your skin or inhaled.

At least 40 oils are used in aromatherapy, categorized according to their effects on the mind, body and specific diseases.

Therapeutic massage may help reduce pain and muscle stiffness and promote relaxation. However, study is needed to determine whether the oils used in aromatherapy provide any additional health benefit.

Biofeedback

This practice uses technology to teach you how to develop certain body responses that help reduce pain. During a biofeedback session, a trained therapist applies electrodes and other sensors to various parts of your body. The electrodes are attached to devices that monitor and give you feedback on body functions, including muscle tension, brain wave activity, respiration, heart rate, blood pressure and temperature.

Once the electrodes are in place, the therapist uses relaxation techniques to calm you, reducing muscle tension and slowing your heart rate and breathing. You then learn how to produce these changes yourself. The goal of biofeedback is to help you enter a relaxed state in which you can better cope with your pain. Sometimes, specific muscle groups are monitored to help you learn how to position yourself in order to reduce muscle strain.

Biofeedback techniques are often taught in physical and occupational therapy or behavioral medicine departments in medical centers and hospitals.

According to a 1995 consensus statement from the NIH, there is evidence that biofeedback can help to relieve many types of chronic pain, including tension headaches and migraines, and pain related to muscle tension.

Chiropractic

Chiropractic medicine is perhaps the most common complementary therapy in the United States. There are two types of chiropractors. Those who depend solely on traditional chiropractic practices are referred to as straight practitioners. Chiropractors who combine standard chiropractic techniques with other therapies, such as exercise, acupuncture or dietary and herbal supplements, are known as mixers.

Chiropractic care has come a long way since the days of its founders, who pointed to misaligned vertebrae as the source of all disease. Today, chiropractors sometimes work with medical doctors as part of the treatment team.

Though they can't prescribe drugs or perform surgery, chiropractors may use some standard medical procedures. And the services of chiropractors are sometimes covered by medical insurance.

Most chiropractors use a hands-on type of adjustment called spinal manipulative therapy, or spinal manipulation. According to chiropractic theory, misaligned vertebrae can restrict your spine's range of motion and affect nerves that radiate from your spine. In turn, the organs that depend on those nerves may function improperly or become diseased. Chiropractic adjustments aim to realign your vertebrae, restore range of motion and free up nerve pathways.

People other than chiropractors also do spinal manipulation. Many osteopathic doctors and physical therapists are trained in this treatment.

Studies indicate that spinal manipulation can effectively treat uncomplicated low back pain, especially if the pain has been present for less than 1 month. Some chiropractors hold to the theory that spinal manipulation can treat diseases other than musculoskeletal problems. There's little scientific evidence to support this.

Dietary and herbal remedies

As anyone who's walked through a health food store can attest, the profusion of dietary supplements and herbal remedies is almost overwhelming. Literally thousands of products crowd the shelves, touting all sorts of claims. Three products heavily marketed for pain relief — especially arthritic pain — are:

Dimethyl sulfoxide. Dimethyl sulfoxide (DMSO) is an industrial solvent, similar to turpentine. Some people believe that when it's rubbed into the skin, it can reduce swelling and pain.

Doctors don't recommend this product for pain relief. Industrial-grade DMSO (sold in hardware stores) may contain poisonous contaminants.

Glucosamine and chondroitin. It's thought that these substances may help reduce pain by repairing damaged cartilage in your joints. Found naturally in your body, glucosamine is incorporated into substances that give cartilage its strength and rigidity.

Glucosamine and chondroitin supplements may help maintain existing cartilage and stimulate growth of new cartilage. The NIH is sponsoring a 4-year study that began in 2000 in which glucosamine and chondroitin are being used to treat more than 1,500 people with osteoarthritis of the knee.

Other herbal treatments. Phenylalanine (DLPA) and marijuana also are promoted as ways to relieve pain. However, the current medical literature doesn't support their effectiveness in treating chronic pain.

Evaluating herbal remedies. Unlike medications you receive from your doctor, dietary and herbal products aren't regulated by the Food and Drug Administration (FDA) for effectiveness. Regulations regarding the safety of these products also are different. With prescription drugs, the manufacturer must prove that the benefits of the drug outweigh any safety concerns before the drug is approved for sale. Dietary and herbal supplements, however, are assumed to be safe until proved otherwise. Only when a supplement is found unsafe is it removed from the market. Because these products don't follow the same safety procedures, they can contain toxic substances that may not be listed on the label. In addition, the amount of active ingredient may vary greatly between different brands.

You might consider herbal products to be natural and, therefore, harmless. However, they can have active chemicals that may not safely mix with other medications you're taking. The best advice is to talk with your doctor before taking any dietary supplement or herbal product.

Homeopathic medicine

Homeopathy, developed in the late eighteenth century by Samuel Hahnemann, is based on two premises:

- *The law of similars:* When given to a healthy person in large quantities, some plant, animal and mineral substances produce symptoms of disease. But when given to a sick person with the same symptoms, smaller doses of the same substances can actually treat an underlying disease.
- *The law of infinitesimals:* Substances treat disease most effectively when they are highly diluted, often in distilled water or alcohol.

The law of similars is sometimes stated as "like cures like" — a capsule summary of homeopathy. Vaccination, a conventional practice, is based on a similar concept that injecting a small dose of an infectious agent stimulates the body's immune system to fight diseases caused by that agent.

However, homeopathy in general departs widely from conventional medicine. Modern drug therapy primarily uses substances to reverse symptoms, not produce them.

At the same time, homeopathy offers one benefit for people who want to explore complementary and alternative medicine. While highly diluted substances may not help you, they probably won't harm you, either.

In addition to using such treatments, homeopaths — people who practice homeopathy — may recommend changes in diet, exercise and other health-related behaviors.

Many studies of homeopathy examine whether the benefits claimed for this treatment result from a placebo effect — that is, from the belief of patients and practitioners in the treatment rather than the treatment itself. One analysis of over 100 controlled, randomized studies concluded that this was not true. In other words, homeopathy appeared to have active results that went beyond the placebo effect. However, there is little published evidence that homeopathy can effectively treat specific diseases or conditions.

Humor therapy

The first studies of the effect of humor on the body were conducted in the United States in the 1930s. But it wasn't until 1979 that humor research got a real boost. That's when *Saturday Review* editor Norman Cousins countered a diagnosis of ankylosing spondylitis, a painful and potentially disabling arthritis, with a combination of mainstream medicine and large doses of humor.

Cousins watched videos of *Candid Camera*, as well as Marx Brothers and Three Stooges films. Although his doctors had given him little chance of recovery, within 8 days his pain began to subside, and he returned to work. He documented his recovery in the book *Anatomy of an Illness* and founded the Humor Research Task Force.

Cousins' experience spawned a wealth of humor research. Studies have been designed to see whether humor can promote relaxation, reduce stress and enhance the immune system. There is some evidence that exposure to comedy can have pain-relieving effects. However, the research is inconsistent on this point, and some of the relevant studies were not well designed. More and better research is needed.

Hypnosis

People have been using hypnosis to promote healing since ancient times. However, in the past 50 years, the use of hypnosis has seen a resurgence among physicians, psychologists and other mental health professionals.

Hypnosis produces an induced state of relaxation in which your mind stays narrowly focused and open to suggestion. It's not known how hypnosis works, but experts believe it alters your brain wave patterns in much the same way as other relaxation techniques.

For treatment of chronic pain, you receive suggestions designed to help you decrease your perception of the pain and increase your ability to cope with it. Unlike situations sometimes portrayed in movies and on TV, you can't be forced under hypnosis to do something you normally wouldn't want to do.

The success of hypnosis depends on your understanding of the procedure and your willingness to try it. You need to be strongly motivated to change. About 80 percent of adults can be hypnotized by a trained professional. People who don't want to feel out of control often can't be hypnotized.

Psychiatrists and psychologists occasionally practice hypnosis. You can also undergo hypnosis from a professional hypnotist. Some people eventually develop the skills to hypnotize themselves. Once you're trained in self-hypnosis, you may be able to use this technique to manage your pain.

A 2002 study conducted in Manchester, England, found that hypnotherapy was effective in treating the symptoms associated with irritable bowel syndrome. Another study published in 2001 supported the value of hypnosis for treating cancer pain and nausea. A 1995 consensus statement from the NIH cited strong evidence that hypnosis can reduce pain associated with cancer. NIH panel members also concluded that hypnosis can provide assistance with other conditions that can lead to chronic pain, such as irritable bowel syndrome and tension headache.

Magnet therapy

Most claims regarding the healing power of magnets are from manufacturers of products that contain magnets, such as arm and leg wraps, belts, mattress pads and shoe inserts. The manufacturers claim the products can relieve various health problems, including chronic pain, by stimulating your body's natural electrical field.

Although research may someday find magnet therapy to be beneficial, to date there's no scientific evidence that magnets used in this manner provide any health benefits. And some experts believe inappropriate use of magnets could possibly lead to health problems.

A few medical researchers are exploring the use of magnets as a therapy for some forms of chronic pain. Initial reports suggest some possible benefits, but more study is needed. The research also involves different, more powerful magnets, not common refrigerator magnets sold in stores or found in some products.

Massage

Massage therapy is one of the oldest methods of health care in practice. It involves use of different manipulative techniques to move your body's muscles and soft tissues. Massage therapists primarily use their hands to manipulate muscles and tissues, but sometimes they may use their forearms, elbows or feet.

Massage therapy is based on the belief that when muscles are overworked, waste products can accumulate in the muscle, causing soreness and stiffness. The therapy aims to improve circulation in the muscle, increasing flow of nutrients and eliminating waste products.

Massage therapists claim that their treatment can relieve stress and anxiety, relax your muscles, help relieve headaches, lower blood pressure, improve range of motion in your joints and increase production of your body's natural painkillers.

Studies are still needed to document the effects of massage. Although massage is generally safe, avoid it if you have open sores, acute inflammation or circulatory problems. Generally, a massage should feel good. If it doesn't, speak up promptly.

Meditation

Meditation is a way to calm your mind and body. It originates from various religious and cultural traditions.

During meditation you sit quietly and focus on a simple activity, such as breathing or a simple word or phrase that's repeated many times. With time, you may find that this practice brings a deeply restful state that reduces your stress response.

In this state, your breathing slows, your muscles relax and your brain wave activity reflects a general state of relaxation.

Although meditation sounds simple, learning to control your thoughts isn't as easy as it may seem. The more you practice, though, the less difficult it becomes to hold your concentration without having your mind wander.

There are hundreds of studies published about various forms of meditation — in particular, the relaxation response and Transcendental Meditation. The quality of these studies is uneven, but they do suggest grounds for further research.

Of particular interest in pain management is the mindfulness meditation program developed at the University of Massachusetts Medical Center in 1979 for people with chronic pain. Across the United States, 250 programs have been based on this model. Only a few studies of mindfulness meditation have been published, though they do suggest a useful role for this technique in pain management.

You can learn meditation from a trained instructor or from a psychologist or other mental health professional. Sometimes, meditation is used in conjunction with biofeedback to help promote relaxation.

Movement therapies

Several nontraditional therapies, such as the Feldenkrais and Trager methods, center around the philosophy that, over time, people start moving and holding their bodies in dysfunctional ways. Weaker muscles end up doing the work of stronger muscles, causing stress and tension.

An instructor takes you through a series of specific movements designed to teach you to use your muscles and joints more comfortably and efficiently. The movements are also designed to help you find greater pleasure in, and ease with, your body.

Practitioners claim these therapies can help control pain and promote an overall sense of well-being. Although they appear to be safe, their benefits aren't scientifically supported.

Music therapy

Practitioners of music therapy claim that it can lower stress, reduce symptoms of depression and promote pain relief. Like other forms of relaxation, performing or listening to music may help reduce pain by relieving muscle tension and slowing your breathing.

Music therapy hasn't been extensively researched, and the few published studies yield contradictory findings. However, it poses few risks and is a relatively inexpensive form of therapy.

Several national organizations promote the use of music for health and healing. These organizations have chapters set up across the country. In addition, some medical centers offer music therapy programs.

Naturopathic medicine

This form of medicine utilizes natural therapies, including acupuncture, manipulative therapy, herbal medicines and nutritional therapies. Instead of using traditional medications or surgery to treat illness, naturopathic doctors rely on methods aimed at strengthening your body's natural healing ability.

To become certified, naturopathic physicians go through 4 years of training. Their training, however, is substantially different from that of traditional medical doctors.

Naturopathic physicians claim they can treat the same range of conditions as conventional doctors. However, these claims aren't backed by research.

Osteopathy

Osteopathy is a recognized medical discipline that has much in common with conventional medicine. Similar to traditional physicians, doctors of osteopathy go through rigorous and lengthy training in academic and clinical settings. They're licensed to perform the same therapies and procedures as traditional medical doctors, including surgery and prescribing medications. They may also specialize in various forms of medicine, such as gynecology and cardiology.

One area in which osteopathy differs from conventional medicine is its reliance on manipulation to address joint and spinal problems. Similar in this respect to a chiropractor, an osteopath performs manipulations to try to release pressure in your joints and align your musculoskeletal structure to improve movement and flow of bodily fluids. However, some osteopaths don't rely as heavily on manipulation as others.

Few studies have examined osteopathy as an alternative to conventional medical treatment. In one study, researchers found no difference in results between standard medical care and osteopathic spinal manipulation for low back pain. However, osteopaths used less medication.

Prolotherapy

Prolotherapy — also known as sclerotherapy or proliferant therapy — involves the injection of solutions into ligaments and tendons near the site of chronic joint and low back pain. Proponents of prolotherapy suggest that looseness in the supporting ligaments and tendons around joints causes pain. They contend that injecting solutions that initially cause inflammation leads to the production of collagen — a component of connective tissue — which gives strength to the affected area and reduces the pain. Although prolotherapy has been in use since 1939, there's no strong clinical evidence that it's effective in treating chronic pain.

Rolfing

This therapy uses deep massage to align your body so that all of its components are positioned correctly.

The theory behind Rolfing is that injury or stress causes tissues to adhere in unhealthy ways, interfering with your body's natural movement and producing symptoms such as fatigue and pain. To restore natural alignment, a Rolfing therapist applies deep pressure in an attempt to stretch the tissues and help reposition your muscles and joints.

There are no scientific studies to support Rolfing's benefits. Its deep massage may help reduce stress and tension. However, some people find the procedure painful, and it may worsen chronic pain.

Tai chi

Tai chi (TIE chee), a form of martial arts developed in China, is becoming a popular method for strengthening muscles, improving joint flexibility and reducing stress.

Tai chi involves gentle, deliberate circular movements, combined with deep breathing. As you concentrate on the motions of your body, you develop a feeling of tranquility. For this reason, tai chi is sometimes described as moving meditation. Similar to other forms of Chinese medicine, it's designed to foster the free flow of chi necessary for health.

Research on tai chi has explored its ability to improve balance and reduce the risk of falls in older people. More studies are needed to explore the role of tai chi in managing pain.

You'll find tai chi classes offered in cities throughout the United States. To locate a class in your community, contact your local senior center, YMCA or health club.

Therapeutic touch

Therapeutic touch is closely related to the religious concept of laying on of the hands, where healing power is believed to flow from the healer to the patient. However, therapeutic touch isn't based on a religious concept. Instead, it comes from the idea that your body generates a field of energy. Illness results when there are disturbances in this energy field.

Practitioners of therapeutic touch attempt to get rid of these disturbances by moving their hands back and forth across your body. They also believe that by transferring energy from their hands to your body, they can encourage healing and reduce pain, stress and anxiety.

More study is needed to determine whether therapeutic touch has health benefits.

Yoga

People practice yoga for many reasons. For some, yoga is a spiritual path. For others, yoga is a way to promote physical flexibility, strength and endurance. In either case, you may find that yoga helps you to relax and manage stress.

Americans generally associate the term *yoga* with one particular school of this ancient discipline — hatha yoga. In most cases, hatha yoga combines gentle breathing exercises with movement through a series of postures called asanas.

To be effective, yoga requires training and regular practice. You can find qualified instructors at yoga schools. You can also learn about yoga through books and videotapes. Depending on your type of pain, you may need to modify or avoid some of the yoga postures to prevent excessive stress to your muscles and joints.

There are a few recent studies of yoga in the medical literature. In one study, people who used yoga and relaxation techniques in addition to a wrist splint experienced more relief from carpal tunnel syndrome than people who used the splint alone. In another study, people with osteoarthritis of the hands who took yoga classes improved their finger joint tenderness and range of motion. They also reduced pain.

Five steps in considering any treatment

Do the treatments listed in the previous section work? Several do appear to safely relieve stress and reduce pain. Some of these therapies are gaining acceptance within mainstream medicine. But there are many products and practices that haven't been adequately studied.

Sorting through all of the claims for complementary and alternative techniques can be a challenging task. Use the following suggestions to get past confusion, control your out-of-pocket costs and promote your safety:

1. Gather information about the treatment
The Internet offers an ideal way to keep up with the latest on complementary and alternative treatments — a fast-changing field. If you don't have Internet access at home or work, then contact your local library to see whether it offers Web access to the public.

Begin with Web sites created by major medical centers, national organizations, universities or government agencies. Sites from the United States Government include:

Agency for Healthcare Research and Quality
www.ahrq.gov

National Center for Complementary and Alternative Medicine
www.nccam.nih.gov

National Institutes of Health
www.nih.gov

Office of Dietary Supplements
http://ods.od.nih.gov

Also look to Mayo Clinic for health news and articles on all aspects of health, including pain management:

Mayo Clinic Health Information
www.MayoClinic.com

2. Find and evaluate treatment providers

After gathering information about a treatment, you may decide to find a practitioner who offers it. Of course, you can always find a name in the Yellow Pages. But also check your state government listings for agencies that regulate and license health care providers. These agencies can list names of practitioners in your area. They also offer a way to check credentials.

Professional associations — such as the American Massage Therapy Association, the American Society of Clinical Hypnosis and the American Academy of Medical Acupuncture — offer other useful sources. Many of these associations will provide names of practitioners in your area. To find addresses and phone numbers for these associations, visit the reference desk at your local library or use the Internet to find associations' Web sites.

Whenever possible, talk to people who've received the treatment you're considering and ask about their experience with specific treatment providers. Start by asking friends and family members. Before you get a treatment, call the provider to schedule an informational interview.

There are risks and side effects with many types of treatment, both conventional and unconventional. With any treatment you consider, find out if the benefits outweigh the risks.

3. Consider treatment cost

Many complementary and alternative approaches aren't covered by health insurance. Find out exactly how much the treatment will cost. Whenever possible, get the total amount in writing before you start treatment.

4. Check your attitude

When it comes to complementary and alternative medicine, steer a middle course between uncritical acceptance and outright rejection. Learn to be open-minded and skeptical at the same time. Stay open to various treatments but evaluate them carefully. Also remember that the field is changing. What's alternative today may be well accepted — or discredited — tomorrow.

5. Opt for a combined approach

Research indicates that the most popular use of unconventional medical treatments is to complement rather than replace conventional medical care. Ideally, the various forms of treatment should work together.

You can use complementary and alternative treatments to maintain good health and to relieve some symptoms. But continue to rely on conventional medicine to diagnose a problem and treat the sources of disease. And tell your medical doctor about all of the treatments you get — both conventional and unconventional.

Be sure to seek conventional treatment if you have a sudden, severe or life-threatening health problem. If you break a bone, get injured in a car accident or develop food poisoning, then make the emergency room your first stop.

Also remember a point that applies to health care of any type — there is no substitute for lifestyle. Most practitioners — conventional or complementary and alternative — will tell you that nutrition, exercise, stress management and safety practices are your keys to improved health and longer life.

Chapter 8

Pain centers and clinics

M ajor life changes sometimes require personal guidance. Learning how to manage chronic pain is one instance where one-on-one help may make a difference. If you feel that you might benefit from more individualized care, consider visiting a facility that specializes in pain management. There, you may benefit from the knowledge of professionals who help people deal with chronic pain on a daily basis.

A pain clinic is a facility with one or more physicians who specialize in the treatment of painful conditions, such as back pain or headache. A pain center is a facility with a multidisciplinary group of physicians whose collective expertise allows for the management of a wide variety of pain problems. Pain centers can handle many types of pain, frequently have ongoing research programs and participate in the training of physicians who specialize in pain treatment.

Where to start

In seeking care for your pain, the first step is to obtain the correct diagnosis. You want to make sure that your pain doesn't signal an infection, cancer or other underlying disease. This process usually starts with your primary care physician, who may refer you to one or more specialists. Often a number of diagnostic tests are performed and initial steps are taken to relieve your pain.

If the pain persists and initial treatments don't bring relief, then you may want consider getting care at a pain center or clinic. Physicians there will perform a thorough history and physical exam. Additional diagnostic tests often are performed. These tests may be noninvasive, such as X-rays, or invasive, such as diagnostic nerve blocks. Once a diagnosis is reached, a treatment plan will be proposed. Understand and consider the risks and benefits of any treatment suggested.

Hopefully the treatment will help your pain. Treatments that aren't helpful should be stopped before new ones are tried. If no effective treatment can be found for your pain, there are still ways to help you cope. This process is called pain rehabilitation. Pain rehabilitation programs help you get the most out of life even if you have unrelieved chronic pain.

Pain rehabilitation programs

Pain rehabilitation programs support the belief that chronic pain affects many aspects of your life and, therefore, requires a broad treatment approach. These programs explore various ways to help you control your pain. In the process, they also help you identify factors in your life that may contribute to your pain or make it more difficult to manage. Often, but not always, pain rehabilitation programs are associated with medical schools or large medical centers.

In many pain rehabilitation programs, pain specialists integrate behavioral and lifestyle changes with physical and occupational therapy and selective use of medications or injections. Depending on the location or cause of your pain, other therapies, such as biofeedback or transcutaneous electronic nerve stimulation (TENS), also may be incorporated into your treatment plan.

The pain management team

The staff members who make up pain rehabilitation programs vary. But most programs include some or all of these key professionals:

Physicians. A doctor who has extensive training and experience in treating chronic pain typically heads up the team. This person may be a family practitioner or have trained in one of several medical specialties, such as neurology, psychiatry, anesthesiology or physiatry (physical medicine and rehabilitation). Just one doctor or a group of doctors may work at the center or clinic.

Psychologists. Psychologists help sort through and address the many behavioral and emotional issues that can accompany chronic pain, such as depression, anger and fear. They also help pinpoint issues that may be contributing to your pain, such as strained relations with family members or stress at work. In addition, psychologists teach important skills such as stress reduction and relaxation techniques.

Nurses. Nurses help monitor medication use or medication withdrawal. They provide information on various treatments and monitor your progress. In many programs, a nurse acts as a case manager, serving as an advocate for you and your family and acting as an intermediary to other professionals on the team. A nurse may be the team member with whom you interact most often.

Physical and occupational therapists. Therapists are vital to the task of rebuilding your strength, endurance and confidence in your ability to function in everyday life.

Physical therapists do this through individualized instruction for a complete fitness program. Occupational therapists bolster your independence by focusing on increasing competency in specific day-to-day tasks. Instruction on proper body mechanics and self-care for sore muscles and stiff joints also are goals of physical and occupational therapy.

Others. Additional professionals who may be part of the pain team include:

- A registered dietitian to help you learn to eat a more nutritious diet and control your weight
- A social worker to help you deal with financial, work, educational or family concerns
- A vocational counselor to help you develop the skills you need to return to work or keep your job
- A recreational therapist to help you safely take part in various recreational activities
- A chaplain to assist with religious and family issues

What to expect

Not all pain rehabilitation programs operate in exactly the same way, but their approach is often quite similar.

Once you've been admitted, you'll receive a thorough evaluation. This may include having staff members review your physical and psychological condition, your use of medication, your work situation and your relationship with your family. The evaluation helps staff devise a treatment plan and goals that address your specific needs. These goals might include helping you get off your medication, return to work, become more physically active and learn to relax.

In some programs, the therapy and attention you receive are intensive. You spend most of your day at the center for about 2 to 4 weeks. During this time you work with physical and occupational therapists and spend time in group sessions. You also meet regularly with your case manager to discuss your progress and any areas that remain difficult for you.

With other programs, the schedule is more relaxed. You meet for just a few hours each week over several weeks.

How to locate a pain facility

To find a reputable pain program that fits your needs, talk with your doctor. Some programs require a letter of referral from your doctor and a copy of your medical records.

If you have a medical school nearby, check to see if it operates a pain center or clinic. Or if you're attending a support group, you can ask members of the group if they've been to a pain facility and listen to what they have to say about that program.

You also can obtain a list of approved pain centers from the Commission on Accreditation of Rehabilitation Facilities. This organization certifies pain rehabilitation centers. Other organizations that you can contact for references include the American Pain Society and the American Academy of Pain Medicine (see "Additional resources" on page 191).

What to look for

Pain centers and pain clinics abound. But because facilities and personnel vary in their qualifications and specialties, consider these factors when evaluating your options:

- **What are the goals of the program?** Is the program focused strictly on relieving your pain? Or does it include services to help determine the cause of your pain or the personal problems that may be associated with your pain?
- **What methods does the program advocate?** Be particularly careful in evaluating programs that advocate long-term use of potentially addictive drugs, such as opioids, or that routinely include surgery or rely on unproven therapies, such as homeopathy or herbal supplements.
- **Are staff members friendly and willing to listen?** It's important that you feel comfortable with those around you. Members of the staff should be interested in you and your condition and take time to listen to your concerns.
- **Is the program accredited or certified?** Pain centers or clinics don't have to be accredited or certified to operate. However, some states require accreditation for insurance reimbursement. Certification also helps ensure that the program meets the basic requirements for appropriate medical care.
- **Does it have a good success rate?** Ask what the long-term success rate of the program is. No program can offer a 100 percent success rate. However, generally about half of the people who visit comprehensive pain centers are able to return to work.
- **Does it include follow-up services?** If you need additional care once you've completed your treatment, there should be a phone number to call or person to contact. Avoid programs that offer no follow-up care.
- **How much does it cost?** Make sure that you know approximately how much the treatment will cost before you start. Check with your insurance company to see what expenses are covered. Some insurance companies cover treatment provided by comprehensive pain programs, while others don't.

Inpatient or outpatient?

When selecting a pain rehabilitation program you may need to consider whether you want to take part in the program as an outpatient, or as an inpatient — staying at the facility during the entire course of your treatment. Both approaches have inherent benefits and disadvantages.

The inpatient approach may be beneficial because you're with staff members who can keep a lookout for your negative pain behaviors and help you work on them in a constructive way. The extra support an inpatient clinic offers also may be advantageous if you need to wean yourself from addictive medications.

However, because of this intense, 24-hour-a-day approach, inpatient pain programs generally are more expensive than outpatient programs.

An outpatient pain center provides most or all of the services as an inpatient program. But you spend nights and weekends at home or elsewhere.

An advantage of outpatient programs is that the cost is usually less. They also allow for time to be with family or at work. However, outpatient programs often last longer than inpatient programs. And if you don't live close to the facility, you may need to arrange for overnight accommodations.

Sometimes, people with an addiction to painkilling medications start out in an inpatient facility and then transfer to an outpatient program to continue treatment.

Your role

Pain centers and clinics are similar to many things in life — you get from the program what you're willing to put into it. If you're unwilling to learn new skills and continue to have a negative attitude, the program may help you very little. But if you enter the program with a positive attitude and realistic expectations, you can come away with a better understanding of what you need to do to manage your pain and confidence in your ability to do it.

Part 3

Managing chronic pain

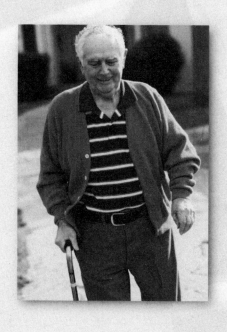

Chapter 9

Taking control of your pain

Many people with chronic pain enjoy active and productive lives. If you aren't among them, there's no reason you can't be. But it's up to you to make it happen.

There aren't any quick fixes for chronic pain. And often, there's only so much doctors can do. You are the key ingredient. If you want your life to improve, you need to lead the way.

You may not like the fact that you have chronic pain. No one does. But clinging to unrealistic hopes or expectations will only prolong your frustration and contribute to your feelings of helplessness.

Understanding your role

The first and most important step in controlling your pain is accepting the fact that you may always have pain. Some people are able to significantly reduce or eliminate their pain. But for most people with chronic pain, it will always be a part of their life.

Managing chronic pain isn't about making your pain disappear. It's about learning how to keep your pain at a tolerable level. It's about enjoying life again, despite your pain. And it's about accepting that only you can control your future.

The choice is yours to make. You can continue to put up with your pain, or you can do something about it. You can dwell on your discomfort, or you can look for solutions.

This can be frightening. For months or even years you may have pinned your hopes on others to treat your condition or tell you what to do. But just as you've learned how to manage other things in your life — your finances, your job and your relationships — you can learn to manage your pain.

The remainder of this book focuses on specific lifestyle issues and pain management strategies that can help you better understand and manage your pain. Each small step you take in your new role as pain manager will boost your self-confidence and strengthen your faith in your abilities.

Finding the right doctor

Being in charge of your pain doesn't mean that you shouldn't seek help from others. Having people who can help you when you have questions or need assistance is important. A doctor can be especially helpful. But make sure it's a doctor who understands your condition and believes in what you're doing.

The right doctor for you could be your family physician or a specialist who's overseeing your condition. Or you may want to see a doctor or a psychologist who specializes in pain management. If you're not sure where to find a pain specialist, ask your doctor to refer you to one. Before selecting a new doctor, however, check with your health insurance provider to make sure that the care will be covered under your policy.

When selecting a doctor, look for someone who:
- Is knowledgeable about chronic pain
- Wants to help
- Listens well
- Makes you feel at ease
- Encourages you to ask questions
- Seems honest and trustworthy
- Allows you to disagree
- Is willing to talk with your family or friends

In addition to finding the right doctor, make an effort to learn all that you can about your condition and your pain. This will make it easier for the two of you to work together as a team.

Where to get more information

Many places offer information about chronic pain or your specific medical condition. Reference areas at most libraries include medical dictionaries, books on health topics and health magazines. You can also browse through the health section at your local bookstore.

Many medical centers, government agencies, nonprofit health organizations and publishers use the World Wide Web as a fast and easy way to provide in-depth health information. If you don't have Internet access, then contact your local public library to see whether it offers access.

But be cautious about what you read or purchase. Just because something has been published, whether in print or on the Web, is no guarantee that the information is accurate or reliable. Anyone who has the necessary hardware and software can publish a Web page and offer medical advice. And just because a Web site looks authoritative doesn't mean it is.

Use reliable sources for your health information. Is it from a respected publication or organization? Has it been reviewed by health professionals? Is it current?

To help you get started, in the back of this book is a list of organizations you can call, write or access via your computer for more information on chronic pain (see "Additional resources" on pages 191 to 194).

Caution: It's important to be informed about your health. However, spending too much time reading about your condition or discussing your pain can be counterproductive. It can draw your attention to your pain, instead of away from it.

Keeping a journal

As you learn techniques to manage your pain, you should see an increase in your activity level and, perhaps, a decrease in your pain level. A daily journal helps you track your progress and determine the therapies or activities that seem to be helping you the most.

A journal is also a way to track goals you want to achieve and your progress in reaching them (see "Sample journal" on page 106).

Many people think that their pain isn't influenced by factors such as work, stress, sleep or physical activity. But after a few months of tracking their pain levels and their activities, they begin to notice some common patterns.

In addition, a journal can be a great way to express your feelings about your pain or other things that are happening in your life. Writing your thoughts and feelings on paper helps you organize and sort through problems and emotions and get them off your chest, similar to the way you feel after a good heart-to-heart visit with a friend or family member.

Pain level and activities

Health care professionals typically measure pain on a scale of 0 to 10, with 0 being no pain and 10 being the worst pain imaginable (see "Rating your pain" on page 105). Using this scale as your guide, a couple of times a day rate your pain level and record it in your journal. In addition, briefly note what you were doing at that time of day.

You can do this whenever it's convenient, but keep the times consistent. Many people choose to record their pain level in the morning when they wake up, after lunch and in the evening before bed.

Keeping a log of your pain levels and activities allows you to:

Learn your pain pattern. Most people find that the changes in their pain levels are quite consistent. For example, your pain may generally be at its lowest level in the morning and its highest level in the evening. Recording your pain levels helps you determine your pain pattern.

Link your pain with your activities. If your pain is always the worst in the evening, why? Look to see if certain activities seem to correlate with an increase or a decrease in your pain level. Are you sitting or standing too long? Is your rush to get dinner ready a contributing factor? Or are you just tired?

Identify flares. Recording your pain levels helps draw attention to inconsistencies. If your pain level at noon is normally a 3 and one day it's a 6, seeing the difference may prompt you to think about your morning. Did you do something different? Did you have an especially stressful morning?

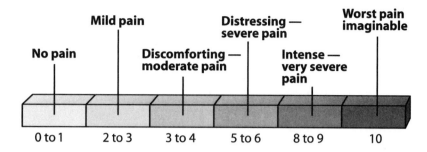

No pain   **Mild pain**   **Discomforting —
moderate pain**   **Distressing —
severe pain**   **Intense —
very severe
pain**   **Worst pain
imaginable**

| 0 to 1 | 2 to 3 | 3 to 4 | 5 to 6 | 8 to 9 | 10 |

Use this scale as a guide when determining your level of pain.

See your progress. If you feel you aren't making progress, reading your journal may help you to realize that your life has improved, even though the process may seem slow. Your journal may also give you clues about why some areas remain difficult for you.

Mood

On a scale of 0 to 10, with 0 being poor and 10 being excellent, rate your mood. This exercise helps you realize that even though your pain and your mood are closely aligned, they aren't bound together.

Typically, the worse your pain, the worse your mood, and vice versa. However, as you begin to feel more in control of your pain, you may find your mood improving at a faster rate than the improvement in your pain levels. Rating your mood helps you realize that even though you may not be able to eliminate your pain, you can learn to live with it and still be happy.

Sleep

A good night's sleep better equips you to handle your day. However, getting enough sleep can be difficult because your pain may keep you up at night. In contrast, some people spend too much time in bed. This can also reduce your pain tolerance.

Once a day, record how many hours you slept during the past 24 hours. Eight hours is average, but the amount of sleep each person needs varies. Your goal should be to feel rested when you wake up.

The importance of sleep and tips to help you sleep better are discussed in Chapter 15.

Sample journal

There is no right or wrong way when it comes to keeping a journal. Some people simply like to jot down their thoughts, and others prefer a worksheet format. This is just one example of how your journal might look and the information to include.

Date: January 1   Hours slept: 7

	7:00 a.m.	1:00 p.m.	10:00 p.m.
Pain level	5	4	6
Mood	7	6	4

Morning

5:00-5:30 Coffee and breakfast
5:30-7:00 Exercised and got ready for work
7:30-11:00 Work
11:30-12:30 15-minute walk and lunch

Afternoon and evening

12:30-4:30 Work
5:00-5:30 Read paper and went through mail
5:30-6:00 Relaxation exercises
6:00-7:00 Dinner
7:00-8:30 Did errands and attended meeting
9:00-10:00 Wrote in journal and got ready for bed.

Comments/thoughts: I slept a little better last night. I still woke up at 5:00 but I didn't feel so tired. I also seem to have more energy at work. I think the morning exercises are helping. Evenings are still a problem. I know I need to rest more but it seems there are just too many things to do.

Setting SMART goals

When you're in pain, it's easy for the pain to become the center of your attention. Things in life that were important to you, or that you were trying to achieve, may take a back seat to the pain.

Setting goals helps divert your attention from your pain and provides an opportunity to think about your lifestyle, and what you can do to better manage your pain. Goals also give you something to strive for.

But goal setting isn't as easy as it may sound. You simply can't identify a couple of things you want and expect them to occur. You'll only be setting yourself up for disappointment.

The key is to set goals that are **specific, measurable, attainable, realistic** and **trackable** (SMART):

Specific. State exactly what you want to achieve, how you're going to do it and when you want to achieve it. To begin with, set goals that you can achieve within a week to a month. It's easy to give up on goals that take too long to reach.

If you have a big goal, break it down into a series of smaller weekly or daily goals. After you achieve one of the smaller goals, move on to the next.

Measurable. A goal doesn't do you any good if there's no way of telling whether you've achieved it. "I want to feel better" isn't a very good goal because it's not specific and it's difficult to measure. "I want to work 8 hours each day" is a better goal because it's specific and measurable.

Attainable. Ask yourself whether the goal is within reasonable reach. For instance, completing a marathon may not be an achievable goal if you've never run before. However, completing a 5K run may be attainable.

Realistic. Is the goal realistic for you? The purpose of a goal is to shift your focus from your pain to your future. But you can't ignore your limitations. Your goals need to be within your capabilities. If you've suffered a serious back injury, a goal of returning to work as a bricklayer may not be realistic. Instead, your goal might be to find a sales job in a related field. Or you might decide to go back to school for training in a new field.

Trackable. Being able to track your progress encourages you to keep going and reach your goal. Look for ways to chart your improvements.

Here's how

These are examples of goals that follow the SMART formula:

Goal: Reduce my use of over-the-counter pain medications
When I want to achieve it: 2 weeks
How I'm going to do it: Plan my day to include exercise, pace myself at work and take frequent breaks, use relaxation techniques
How I'm going to measure it: Each day, record in my journal the medication I took and how much

Goal: Exercise 40 minutes each day
When I want to achieve it: 4 weeks
How I'm going to do it: Stretch and do strengthening exercises 15 minutes in the morning, walk 10 minutes during my lunch hour, bicycle 15 minutes in the evening
How I'm going to measure it: Record in my journal when I exercised and for how long

Consider setting goals for yourself in the following areas:
- Physical activity
- Emotions and behavior
- Stress and relaxation
- Family and friends
- Leisure and recreation
- Work
- Medication
- Spirituality

Your turn

Think carefully about some short-term or long-term goals you want to achieve. If you have some in mind, write them down now.

Chapter 10

Get moving with exercise

There was a time when people with chronic pain were told to avoid physical activity for fear it would damage their joints and muscles and worsen their pain. No more.

When you aren't active, you begin to lose muscle tone and strength and your cardiovascular system works less efficiently. Inactivity also increases your risk of high blood pressure, high cholesterol and diabetes, putting you at increased risk of heart attack and stroke. In addition, inactivity can increase fatigue, stress and anxiety — as well as your pain.

A common misconception is that exercise aggravates pain. On the contrary, exercise can help reduce it. During physical activity, your body releases chemicals (endorphins and enkephalins) that block pain signals from reaching your brain. These chemicals also help alleviate anxiety and depression, conditions that can make your pain more difficult to control.

A regular exercise program that includes flexibility, aerobic and strengthening exercises can help improve your fitness and control your pain. You may feel that you're out of shape or too old to benefit from an exercise program, but it's never too late. Studies have shown that people in their nineties can add muscle mass, become more flexible and increase their aerobic capacity when they start exercising regularly.

Regular exercise also:
- Gives you energy and improves sleep.
- Promotes weight loss, reducing stress on your joints.
- Increases bone mass, reducing your risk of injury.

To help you get and stay active, here's a fitness program that's safe for almost anyone. To benefit from the program, try to exercise most, if not all, days each week.

Before you get started

It's always a good idea to talk with your doctor before starting any type of physical activity program. If you have another health problem or you're at risk for cardiovascular disease, you may need to take some precautions while you exercise.

It's especially important that you see your doctor if you:
- Have a blood pressure of 160/100 mm Hg or higher
- Have diabetes or heart, lung or kidney disease
- Are a man age 40 or older or a women age 50 or older and haven't had a recent physical examination
- Have a family history of heart-related problems before age 55
- Are unsure of your health status
- Have previously experienced chest discomfort, shortness of breath or dizziness during exercise or strenuous activity

---

Improving flexibility

Flexibility exercises include simple range-of-motion and stretching exercises. These exercises ease movement in your joints, allowing you to move and carry out daily activities more comfortably. They also prevent your muscles from shortening and tightening, which can in turn increase your risk of injury.

Range-of-motion exercises
Include some or all of the exercises on the following pages in your physical activity program. With each exercise, move slowly and easily.

Neck

- Bring your chin toward your chest. Then return to normal position. Avoid extending your neck too far back as this can worsen neck pain.
- Tilt your left ear toward your left shoulder. Then return to normal position and tilt your right ear toward your right shoulder. Avoid raising your shoulder toward your head.
- Turn your face to the left, then to the right. Keep your neck, shoulders and trunk straight.

Jaw

- Open your mouth as wide as possible without clicking or popping. Close.
- Move your jaw to the right, then to the left.
- Move your jaw forward, then back.

Shoulders

With your arms at your sides:
- Roll your shoulders forward in a circular motion. Reverse.
- Bring your arms forward and over your head. Keep your trunk straight.
- Raise your arms from your sides to over your head. Keep your trunk straight and your palms up.
- Bring your elbows to shoulder height. Pull your elbows backward and feel a stretch in your chest muscles.

Elbows

- Bend and straighten your elbows.
- Keeping your arms next to your body, bend your elbows to make a right angle and turn your palms up and down.

Wrists

- Move your hands from side to side as far as possible, bending at the wrists.
- Move your hands up and down as far as possible, bending at the wrists.

Fingers and thumbs

- Bend your fingers to make a fist. Then fully straighten them.
- Bend your fingers at the knuckles, forming a claw. Then straighten them.
- Bend your thumbs across your palms and pull toward your little fingers.
- Touch the tips of your thumbs to the tips of your little fingers. Open your hands wide. Repeat, touching your thumb to each finger.

Hips

- March in place, bringing your knees up high.
- Raise your leg out to the side. Alternate legs.
- Lift your leg backwards, keeping your knee straight. Don't arch your back. Alternate legs.
- Kick your feet up behind you by bending your knees.

Trunk

Standing with your hands on your hips:

- Bend your upper body to the left. Repeat to the right.
- Twist your upper body to the right. Repeat to the left. Don't turn your pelvis.

Ankles and feet

Standing with your feet about 12 inches apart:

- Rise on the toes of both your feet. Relax to starting position. Rise on the toes of your right foot. Relax. Rise on the toes of both feet. Relax. Rise on the toes of your left foot. Relax.
- Walk on your heels.
- Walk on your toes.
- Walk heel-to-toe, as though you're on a tightrope.

Stretching exercises

Stretching each time you exercise helps keep your muscles limber, reducing tightness in the muscles. Stretch slowly, holding the position for 30 to 60 seconds, and then slowly release. Breathe deeply and slowly while you stretch. Never bounce, and stretch only until you feel a noticeable pull. Your muscles respond to overstretching by tightening — the opposite of what you want.

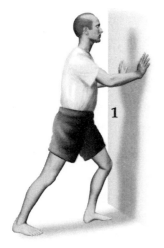

Heel cord stretch (1). Stand at arm's length from a wall with your palms flat against the wall. Keep one leg back with your knee straight and your heel flat on the floor. Slowly bend your elbows and front knee as you lean toward the wall. Hold. Repeat on the other leg.

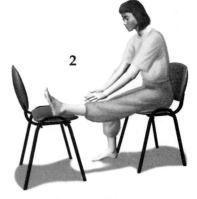

Hamstring stretch (2). Sit on a low table or a chair with your leg propped on another chair in front of you. Without bending your knees, lean forward from your hips. Keep your back straight. Lean forward until you feel a gentle pull in the muscles under your thighs. Hold. Repeat on the other leg.

Quadriceps stretch (3). Stand facing a wall, chair or any other support. Place your left hand against the wall or on the support. Grasp the top of your right foot with your right hand and gently pull your foot or heel up toward your buttocks until you feel mild tension in the front of your thigh. Hold your abdomen in and keep your back straight. Keep the knee of the leg you're stretching directly under you. Relax as you hold the stretch and repeat with the other leg. This exercise may also be done while sitting on the edge of a chair. Consider this if it's difficult for you to balance on one foot.

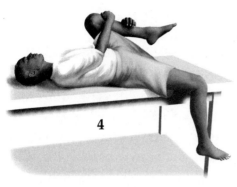

4

Hip flexor stretch (4). Lie on a low table or a bed with your right leg and hip near the edge. Pull your left thigh and knee firmly toward your chest until your lower back flattens against the table or bed. Let your right leg hang in a relaxed position over the edge of the table or bed. Hold. Repeat with the other leg.

Low back stretch (5). Lie flat on a firm surface. With your knees bent, lift one leg at a time toward your body. Grasp your knees and pull toward your shoulders. Stop when you feel a stretch in your lower back. Hold. Return legs, one at a time, to starting position. Repeat. Avoid this exercise if you have osteoporosis or a hip replacement.

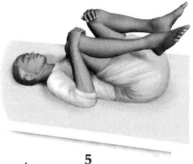

5

Looking for a helping hand?

For help with designing and getting started on your activity program, contact one of these professionals:

Physical therapist. Most hospitals and clinics have physical therapists on staff. A physical therapist is trained in the use of exercise to achieve physical fitness. He or she can help you select the most appropriate exercises based on the location of your pain and show you how to do the exercises properly.

Occupational therapist. Occupational therapists also are available in most hospitals and clinics. An occupational therapist can teach you how to do daily activities in ways that won't place extra stress on your joints.

Certified exercise therapist. Many health clubs have employees who are trained in exercise therapy. If you belong to a health club — or are thinking of joining one — make an appointment to meet with a certified therapist for help with developing an exercise plan.

Increasing aerobic capacity

Aerobic exercises place added demands on your heart, lungs and muscles, increasing your heart rate, blood pressure and need for oxygen. These exercises help your body work more efficiently and reduce your risk of cardiovascular disease, including heart attack, high blood pressure and high cholesterol.

Aerobic activity also increases your stamina so you don't become as easily fatigued and you have more energy for daily activities.

Aim for 20 to 40 minutes of moderately intense aerobic activity most, if not all, days each week. If you've been inactive, start out slowly and at an easy pace and gradually increase your time and level of exertion.

There are many forms of aerobic activity. Walking is the most common because it's easy, convenient and inexpensive. All you need is a good pair of walking shoes.

Other aerobic exercises include:

- Aerobic dance
- Cross-country skiing
- Golfing
- Snowshoeing
- Bicycling
- Dancing
- Hiking
- Swimming and water aerobics

Water aerobics have become increasingly popular among people with chronic pain because water's buoyancy reduces stress on your joints. Water also provides resistance to increase the benefits of aerobic activity. In addition, many people find warm water to be relaxing and soothing to sore muscles and joints.

A disadvantage of water exercises is that they aren't weight-bearing. To maintain bone mass and protect against osteoporosis, combine water exercises with activities such as walking or lifting weights.

Building strength

Strong muscles improve your physical fitness and reduce fatigue. They also make it easier to carry out more vigorous types of daily activities, such as carrying laundry up and down stairs or lifting items at work.

To build muscle, include some or all of these exercises most, if not all, days you exercise. If you're out of shape, begin with 5 repetitions of each and try to build to 25 repetitions.

Abdominal exercises
Lie on the floor or on a table, with your knees bent (6). Raise your head and shoulders so your shoulder blades lift off the floor or table. Try to keep your head in a neutral position. Hold for 1 or 2 seconds. Bring your head and shoulders back down. Repeat, reaching both hands toward your left knee (7). Relax. Repeat, reaching both hands toward your right knee.

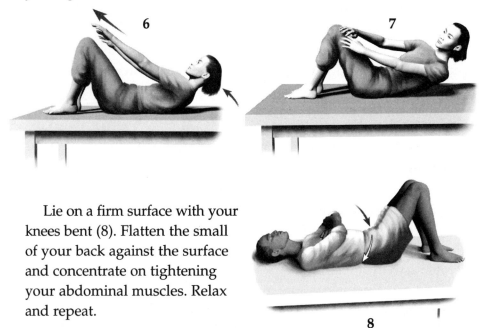

Lie on a firm surface with your knees bent (8). Flatten the small of your back against the surface and concentrate on tightening your abdominal muscles. Relax and repeat.

What about weightlifting?

Lifting weights is an excellent way to strengthen your muscles. However, it's best to work with a physical therapist or fitness trainer in developing and beginning a weightlifting program. A therapist or trainer will help you select the appropriate weights for your level of fitness and teach you how to lift them properly to avoid injury to your muscles and joints.

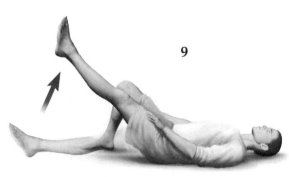

Lie on your back with your right knee bent and your left knee straight (9). Hold your abdominal muscles tight, and slowly lower and raise your left leg. Relax and repeat. Reverse legs. Avoid doing abdominal exercise if you have osteoporosis.

Back exercises

Lie facedown over a large pillow with a folded towel under your forehead. Position the pillow under your belly button to keep your spine in a neutral position (10). Place your hands at your sides. Pulling your shoulder blades together, raise your head and chest. Keep your neck relaxed. Return to the starting position and repeat.

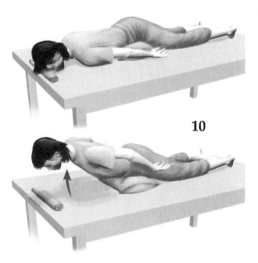

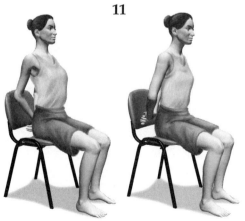

Sit upright in a chair (11). Put your hands on your hips or behind your back, and pull your shoulder blades together. Hold for 5 seconds. Relax and repeat.

Leg exercises

Set up two chairs, one in front of the other (12). Hold on to the back of the chair in front of you and begin to sit in the chair behind you. Partway down, stop and hold your position for 3 to 5 seconds. Return to standing and repeat.

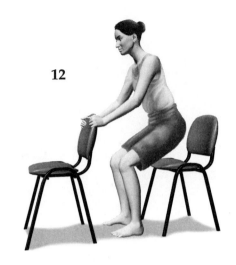

12

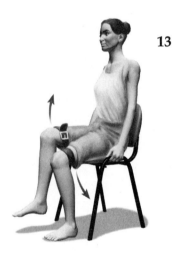

13

Sit back in a chair. Weave a belt around your legs just above your knees so it forms a figure eight (13). Pulling your legs in opposite directions, lift one leg off the floor. Relax. Repeat with other leg.

Sit far back on a table or in a chair. Weave a belt around your ankles so it forms a figure eight (14). Try to straighten one leg while pulling the other foot backward, applying equal force with both legs. Relax. Repeat with the other leg.

14

Chest and arm exercises

Sit in a sturdy chair that has arms (no wheels), with your feet firmly on the floor. Place your hands on the arms. Push your body up off the surface of the chair using your arms only, not your feet (15). Relax.

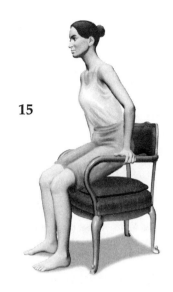

15

16

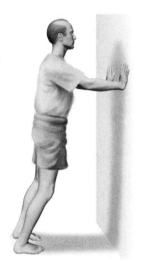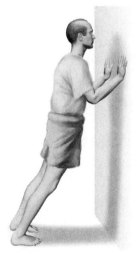

Stand facing a wall, far enough away that you can place your palms on the wall with your elbows slightly bent (16). Slowly bend your elbows and lean toward the wall. Straighten your arms and return to a standing position. Repeat. As you build strength, try standing farther from the wall.

Perfecting your posture

Good posture places only minimal strain on your joints and muscles. Poor posture, however, can increase stress on some muscles, stretching them or causing them to shorten. When overstretched, your muscles lose their strength. Muscles that are too short are less flexible and more prone to injury and pain.

Common forms of poor posture include the swayback posture (left), and slouch posture (right).

Avoid poor posture

One extreme of poor posture is the swayback. In this position your stomach protrudes too far in front and your buttocks extend too far in the rear. Because of this, your backbone takes on an exaggerated curve between your pelvis and your ribs. Swayback posture puts excessive pressure on your lower back and can contribute to back problems.

The opposite extreme is the slouch, in which your shoulders are rolled forward. If you perpetually slouch, muscles in your chest shorten, reducing your flexibility.

Practice good posture

Good posture will help relax your muscles and may reduce your pain. Throughout the day, including while you exercise, try to maintain good posture.

How to straighten up

Here are some tips that can help you improve your posture:

- Sit in a straight-back chair with your back supported.
- Keep your car seat upright so that your hips are at a 90-degree angle.
- Think "tall" when you stand and keep your stomach muscles tight.
- Stand with your weight on both feet.
- Maintain a healthy weight and exercise regularly.
- Sleep on a firm mattress, and use a pillow that comfortably supports your neck.

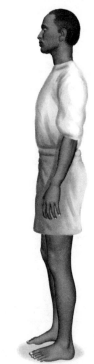

Good standing posture: Head erect with chin tucked in, chest held high, shoulders relaxed, hips level, knees straight but not locked, feet parallel.

- Wear comfortable shoes without high heels.
- Avoid tight pants and belts.
- Don't carry a bag on your shoulder, such as a purse, that weighs more than 2 pounds.

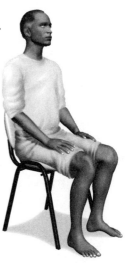

Good sitting posture: Spine and head erect, back and legs at a 90-degree angle, natural curves in back maintained.

Keeping your program on track

Regular exercise and good posture can help you stay active and continue to enjoy your favorite leisure activities. As you become more physically fit, you'll also notice an improvement in your energy level. In addition, many people find that as their fitness improves, so does their mood.

The following suggestions may help you to stay motivated:

Set goals

Start with simple goals and then progress to longer-range goals. People who can stay physically active for 6 months usually end up making regular activity a habit. Remember to make your goals realistic and achievable. It's easy to get frustrated and give up on goals that are too ambitious.

Start slowly

The most common mistakes many people make are starting an exercise program at too high an intensity and progressing too quickly. It's often not until the next day that you discover you've overdone it, and the resulting pain and stiffness can be very discouraging. It's better to progress slowly and stay within your capacity than to push it too fast and be forced to abandon your program because of increased pain.

Add variety

Vary what you do to prevent boredom. For example, try alternating walking and bicycling with swimming or a low-impact aerobic dance class. On days when the weather is pleasant, do your flexibility or stretching exercises outside. Consider joining a health club to broaden your access to different forms of physical activity.

Be flexible

If you're traveling or especially busy on a certain day, it's OK to adapt your exercises to accommodate your schedule. If you develop a cold or the flu, take off a day or two from your exercise program. Fatigue can increase pain.

Track your progress

Record what you do each time you exercise, how long you do it, and how you feel during and after exercising. Recording your efforts helps you work toward your goals and reminds you that you're making progress.

Be social

Exercise with a friend or make new friends who like to exercise by joining a group or taking a class.

Reward yourself

Work on developing an internal reward that comes from feelings of accomplishment, self-esteem and control of your own behavior. After each exercise session, take 2 to 5 minutes to sit down and relax. Savor the good feelings that exercise gives you, and think about what you've just accomplished. This type of internal reward can help you make a long-term commitment to regular exercise.

External rewards can also help keep you motivated. When you reach a longer-range goal, treat yourself to a new pair of walking shoes or a new CD.

Chapter 11

Organizing your day

How you organize and go about your day can significantly affect your ability to manage your pain. If you overdo it to meet a deadline at work or overcommit yourself so that you're running from one activity to the next, your body reaches a point where it can't keep up. Fatigue and frustration set in and your pain increases. This can keep you from doing other things that are equally important, such as spending time with family and friends, or having quiet time for yourself.

The opposite isn't any better — avoiding daily activities and spending hours lying around the house. The isolation that this lifestyle produces can cause you to focus only on your pain.

The answer is a day that includes a healthy balance — time for work, socializing with family and friends, exercise and recreation, hobbies, relaxation and rest. Achieving such a balance can be difficult. Like many people, you may have a lot of commitments and responsibilities. It also isn't easy to change old habits.

Instead of drastically altering your daily routine so that it feels uncomfortable, take it one small step at a time. Each week, try to incorporate several small changes. Over time, you'll achieve the balance that's right for you.

How does your day balance out?

Think of how you spend a typical weekday. Does it include a balance of activities? The first example below shows imbalance. Work consumes most of this person's daytime hours, leaving little time

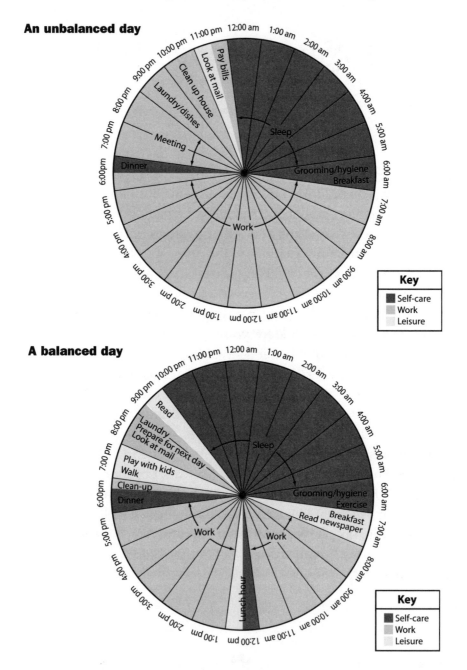

An unbalanced day

Key
■ Self-care
▨ Work
□ Leisure

A balanced day

Key
■ Self-care
▨ Work
□ Leisure

for other activities. The second example shows a balanced day that includes time for exercise and relaxation. A healthy balance includes time for being productive, resting and having fun.

During the week and on the weekends, try not to spend a disproportionate amount of time on any one activity, such as more than 8 hours at work. Instead, aim to include as many activities in your day as feels comfortable — including adequate time for rest.

Putting time on your side

For many people, an important step to balancing their day is learning to use time more efficiently. Juggling work, household tasks and social activities can consume large amounts of your day. Procrastination, perfectionism or overcommitting yourself can make time management even more difficult. Taking charge of your time can have a significant impact on how you feel and how much energy you have.

Try these strategies for using your time more effectively:

Plan. Schedule your day so that you have time for the things you need to do and those you want to do. Write down all of your activities in a daily planner. Then frequently refer to your planner to make sure you stay on track. At the back of this book (see "Your personal planner" on page 181), you'll find a sample planner with some blank pages to get you started.

It may also be helpful to place a calendar near your telephone to mark down all events and appointments so that they don't come as a surprise and to avoid doubling up on commitments. Using a planner doesn't require rigid scheduling. Rather, it simply provides a framework with which you take control of how you spend your time.

Recognize patterns. Notice when you waste time and avoid these time wasters. If you can't avoid them, try to make them productive. For example, while waiting for a doctor's appointment or during your daily train commute, listen to a relaxation tape or balance your checkbook.

Prioritize. If you're involved in many activities that are competing for your time, decide which are the most important and let go of the rest. Be aware that another person's priority doesn't have to be your priority. There are times when your needs come before the needs of others. The consequences of not taking care of yourself likely will be increased pain and fatigue.

Delegate. On days when you have more to do than you can comfortably handle, seek help from others. Asking for assistance, or allowing others to take responsibility for certain things, doesn't indicate a weakness or flaw in your character. On the contrary, delegating is an example of good time and energy management.

Evaluate. Think about your day. Are your expectations regarding the number of tasks you can complete in a day realistic?

Educate. Discuss your time needs with those who rely on you the most. If family members, friends or co-workers make unreasonable demands on your time, explain to them that to stay active and healthy you're learning to pace yourself, and that you must make a conscious effort to live a balanced life.

Getting more organized

Becoming more organized can save you time so that you can incorporate more activities into your day. Organization also helps conserve energy by eliminating wasted steps and unnecessary motions.

Think before you act. Before you begin a task, gather all of the items you need or make a list. For example, keep all of your cleaning supplies in one bucket to avoid multiple trips up and down the stairs. Or list what you need to do before you run errands, to avoid a second trip later on.

Keep commonly used items accessible. Organize your work areas at home and at your job so that items you use frequently are close at hand. This can save you unnecessary bending or reaching. At home, this might include keeping your spoons and spatulas next to the stove or your wrenches and screwdrivers on a pegboard above your workbench. At work, you might keep your phone adjacent to your computer or frequently used files on your desk.

Reduce clutter. Searching for items takes time and energy. Organize your counters, cabinets, closets and drawers so that you can easily find what you need. Don't let housework and paperwork pile up.

Taking everything in moderation

Moderation involves how much, how long or how fast you do things to avoid overdoing or underdoing activities during your day. By moderating activities, you can improve your ability to accomplish daily tasks without increasing pain levels or fatigue.

To practice moderation:

Break apart lengthy tasks. Lengthy activities often deplete your energy and may increase your pain. Instead of spending all day Saturday planting your garden, spend 1 or 2 hours in the garden over 3 or 4 days. Another example is to divide a 10-hour car trip to visit relatives into 2 days instead of 1. Get out and stretch every 90 minutes or 90 miles.

Alternate activities. Mix activities that require a lot of effort with those that require only a little energy. After vacuuming one room of the house, sit down and fold laundry or pay bills. After mowing the lawn, sit down and read or watch a movie.

Prioritize tasks. Note times of the day when you have the most energy and you're feeling your best. Plan your priority tasks during these times.

Take frequent rest breaks. How often you should take a break depends on the activity. You may find you can do some activities, such as word processing, for 30 minutes to an hour before you need a break. More strenuous tasks, such as mowing the lawn, may require a break every 10 to 20 minutes. It's important to take a break before you become fatigued.

Work at a moderate pace. Instead of rushing to complete a task, take your time and work at a comfortable speed — one at which you feel like you're exerting yourself but not overdoing it. You expend twice as much energy when you work at a fast pace compared with a moderate one. It may take you a little longer to get the job done, but in the end you'll feel better.

Change the frequency of tasks. Some tasks may be less fatiguing if you break them up and do them more often. For example, try doing your laundry three times a week with smaller loads rather than spending several hours on one day doing the chore.

Changing how you do things

Do you always stand at the kitchen counter while chopping vegetables? Do you balance on your tiptoes and stretch your arm to reach items on high shelves? Do you sit while reading through correspondence at work? If so, do you know why? Chances are, your answer is "That's the way I've always done it."

Adding balance to your day also involves looking for new and more efficient ways to perform everyday tasks. You want to avoid reaching, bending, twisting or prolonged sitting or standing, actions that consume energy and that can aggravate your pain. Instead of standing to cut vegetables, pull up a stool or take the vegetables and cutting board with you and sit at the kitchen table. Instead of stretching to reach an item, use a footstool. Instead of always sitting at your desk, walk around your office while you read.

The less tired you are from doing simple things, the more energy you'll have for more strenuous tasks. Here are examples of some simple ways you can modify your day.

While getting dressed
- Gather all articles of clothing.
- Sit down to put on your clothes.
- Place your foot on a chair or stool when tying your shoes.
- Avoid clothes that button or tie in the back.

In the kitchen
- Bend your knees, not your back, to reach items on lower shelves.
- Place one foot on a footstool when standing for long periods, and alternate feet. Whenever possible, sit down.
- Organize cupboards to keep frequently used items within easy reach
- Store heavy items within easy reach — at hip to chest level.
- Use electrical appliances when possible, such as an electric can opener, mixer and knife.
- Choose quick and easy recipes or double recipes and freeze extra portions for another day's meal.

Around the house

- Use a long-handled duster for hard-to-reach corners and a long-handled mop to clean your floors.
- Use your legs, not your arm, to move the vacuum cleaner.
- Sit on a stool to remove laundry from your dryer.
- Position your bed so that you have access to it from three sides. When making your bed, get on your knees to tuck in bed sheets and blankets. Instead of lifting the mattress, push the sheets and blankets between the mattress and box spring.

When outdoors

- Use a wheeled cart to move heavy items.
- Mow your lawn with a self-propelled mower.
- Purchase power tools, such as a nail driver and screwdriver.
- Use a long-handled rake or hoe to avoid bending.
- Bend your knees when shoveling snow, and use your legs to lift the load. Use a small, lightweight shovel. Slide the snow as much as possible.

Moving your body wisely

Changing how you perform daily activities is based on using your muscles and joints correctly. Proper body mechanics begin with good posture. When you stand or sit, try to keep your shoulders and neck relaxed and your spine aligned properly.

If you sit for prolonged periods, occasionally elevate your legs by placing your feet on a footstool. Also change positions to shift your weight. This helps divert stress to different muscles.

The same strategies apply to prolonged standing. Shift your weight to change positions and use a low footstool. Place one foot on the stool and frequently alternate your feet. For both sitting and standing, take a 5- to 10-minute break every 30 to 60 minutes.

Here are other examples of proper ways to move.

Reaching

- Avoid excessive arching and twisting of your back.
- Maintain normal spine curves.

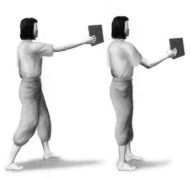

• Place one foot forward as close to the object as possible. Grasp the object and pull it slowly to the edge of the shelf by shifting your body weight to your back foot.
• Slowly lower the object to waist level, using your arms. Keep the object as close to you as possible.

Kneeling

• Keep your feet 8 to 12 inches apart.
• Place one foot forward, and lower your body down to one knee by bending at the hips and knees, keeping your body weight on the balls of your feet.

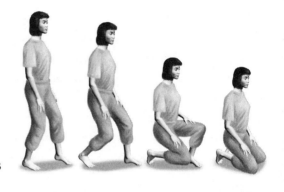

• If you need, use your arms to help you move in and out of a kneeling position.

Don't hold your breath

If you've been in an exercise class, you may have heard your instructor say, "Don't forget to breathe." And you may have said to yourself, "Of course I'm breathing."

It's common to hold your breath when you're concentrating on an activity, such as exercising, or struggling with a simple task, such as opening a lid on a jar. And often, you don't even realize that you're doing it. When you hold your breath, however, you limit oxygen to your muscles just when they need it the most. Because your muscles can't perform to their capacity without adequate oxygen, you become more easily fatigued.

To keep from holding your breath, exhale when you exert the most energy, such as twisting a jar lid or lifting a heavy box from the floor. Your body will naturally respond by breathing in.

- Maintain normal spine curves.
- To progress to full kneeling, lower yourself until both knees are on the floor, and sit back on your heels.
- Reverse the process to stand.

Lifting

- Follow the steps for kneeling, making sure you stand close to the object you're going to lift.
- If the object is heavy, lift it first to your bent knee.
- Lift using your leg muscles to rise from the floor.
- Carry the object close to your body at about waist level. If possible, place your forearms under the object.
- Turn by pivoting your feet. Don't twist at your waist.

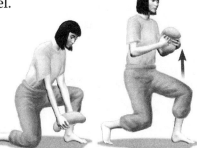

Pushing

- Bend your knees so that your arms are level with the object.
- Maintain normal spine curves and walk, using your legs to push the object ahead of you.

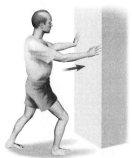

Pulling

- Bend your knees so that your arms are level with the object.
- Maintain normal spine curves and walk backward, pulling the object with your whole body weight instead of just your arms or back.
- If possible, push rather than pull.

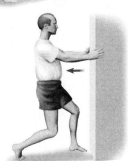

Using long-handled tools

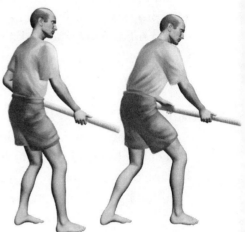

- Stand with one foot forward. Use a rocking motion. With the forward stroke, shift your body weight to your forward foot. When you pull back, shift your weight to your back foot.
- Use arm and leg movements instead of back movements.
- Avoid overreaching and twisting. Use long, smooth strokes.
- Occasionally switch hand positions, exchanging your top hand with your bottom hand.

Avoiding temperature extremes

Controlling your exposure to extreme heat or cold also can help reduce fatigue. If you need to be outside in hot weather, complete your activities in the morning when heat and humidity may be less. Wear a hat or cap and light-colored clothing to reflect the sun's rays, and if possible, work in an area where there's shade or a breeze.

In cold weather, dress warmly and wear a hat or cap to prevent loss of body heat. Wear several layers of clothing so that you can add or remove layers as needed to maintain a comfortable body temperature.

Chapter 12

Dealing with your emotions and behaviors

When chronic pain intrudes on your life, you may find yourself overwhelmed by intense, often negative, emotions, including panic, fear, grief and anger. Like the pain that causes them, these emotions can linger and transform you into a different person — a person you don't like.

Changes in your behavior, expressed through words and actions, can affect your sense of self-worth and your relationships. These changes can also affect your body, sapping your energy and intensifying your pain.

But there are positive ways for dealing with these changes. The techniques outlined in this chapter are designed to help you recognize and deal with negative changes, improve relationships and become more effective at managing your pain.

Admitting your loss

For many people, the first step in dealing with negative feelings is to admit that the feelings exist. That's very difficult for some people to do, especially in a culture that often praises the optimist and criticizes the complainer.

If you're grappling with chronic pain, one of the earliest and most wrenching emotions you experience is a deep sense of loss.

You may miss:

- The healthy person you once were
- Your independence
- Your privacy
- Job satisfaction
- An enjoyable hobby
- Sexual intimacy
- Untroubled family relationships
- Gatherings with friends
- Feelings of energy and confidence
- A sense of happiness

These are difficult losses. You may feel as if you've lost nearly everything precious to you. Your natural response is to grieve.

Feelings associated with grieving

Grieving can trigger various feelings. Many people respond to chronic pain with the same feelings that often accompany loss of a loved one.

Denial. You may deny you're in pain. You continually seek a cure even though you've been told your pain is incurable.

Anger or frustration. You've tried numerous ways to control your pain, and nothing seems to be working. You find yourself more irritable more often. You get upset because others don't seem to understand what you're going through.

Depression. You become overwhelmed by feelings of sadness, worthlessness and helplessness. You don't feel like doing anything, and you have difficulty concentrating. You withdraw from others.

Guilt and shame. You sense you're not the person you used to be. You feel you're letting down those who are closest to you.

Acceptance. You stop focusing on things you can't change and begin to look to the future. You accept that your pain is a part of your life.

As you work your way through these emotions, consider these suggestions:

- Recognize your losses as serious. Don't trivialize them.
- Admit your feelings to yourself and others — especially supportive family, friends and your doctor. Acknowledging and talking about your feelings is the first step toward emotional health.
- Give yourself time for emotional healing, and ask your doctor, a counselor or a therapist for advice and help.

Managing your anger

Unrelenting pain, interrupted sleep, unsuccessful treatments, job difficulties and insurance battles — there are a lot of things that can make you angry when you're experiencing pain. But it's unhealthy to stay angry, bottle up your anger or express it with explosive outbursts.

Mismanaged anger can hurt you in many ways. Whether it's short-term and intense or lingering and subdued, anger can lead to headaches, backaches, high blood pressure, irritable bowel syndrome and other health problems. Anger also can influence your pain. It typically produces muscle tension, making it difficult to relax.

Here are some ideas to help you manage your anger:

Identify your anger triggers. If, for example, you know ahead of time that a visiting friend generally manages to upset you, you can prepare for the next visit. Think about topics that spark your anger, and practice what to say to defuse the situation. For example, if your friend starts to bring up a past dispute, you might respond by saying, "Oh, we've discussed that before. Certainly we've got more interesting things to talk about."

Identify symptoms of emerging anger. What do you do when you start to get angry? Do you clench your teeth? Do your neck and shoulders begin to tense up? Read these symptoms like a caution light — a warning that you're getting angry.

Respond to your symptoms. When you find yourself becoming angry, take a short timeout. Count to 10, take a few deep breaths, look out a window — anything to buy time so that your brain can catch up with your emotions, and you can think before you act.

Give yourself time to cool down. Before you confront the person who has made you angry, find a way to release some of your emotional energy. Go for a walk, run or clean the house.

Don't bottle up your anger. If your anger stems from what someone did or said, talk directly to that person. Don't verbally attack the person with accusations and a history of how this person has angered you in the past. Deal only with this episode, and approach it from the perspective of how you feel instead of what the person did. For example, try a statement like this: "I feel hurt by what you said." That way, you're more likely to find a receptive listener than if you launch a blame-offensive statement, such as, "You insulted me for the 20th time today!"

Find release valves. Look for creative ways to release the energy produced by your anger. These might include listening to music, painting or writing in your journal.

Seek advice. If anger-provoking situations continue, confide in people who care about you, such as a family member or friend. Ask them to help you brainstorm possible solutions. You might even try role-playing scenes that spark your anger so that you can practice a healthy response.

You can't keep yourself from getting angry, but you can manage your anger so that it doesn't become an ongoing problem that aggravates your pain.

Managing your fear and anxiety

When you have chronic pain, you may fear the worst. You may worry about re-injury, changes in finances, job status and increased pain. Such fears contribute to self-limiting behavior and a self-defeating attitude. Instead, practice positive self-talk and try to objectively examine the cause of your fears. Talk with your doctor about fears related to your symptoms. Set realistic goals and expectations for yourself. If anxiety interferes with your daily functioning, seek professional advice and counseling.

Practicing positive thinking

There are many ways to cope with the upsetting changes and emotions chronic pain can produce. One coping technique is positive self-talk. Self-talk is the stream of thoughts that run through your head every day. Some people refer to this as automatic thinking.

Your automatic thoughts may be positive or negative. Some are based on logic and reason. Others may be misconceptions that you formulate from lack of adequate information. The goal of positive self-talk is to weed out the misconceptions and challenge them with rational and positive thoughts.

Learning positive self-talk

The process is simple, but it takes time and practice. Throughout the day, stop and evaluate what you're thinking and find a way to put a positive spin on negative thoughts. Don't say to yourself anything you wouldn't say to someone else. If a negative thought enters your mind, evaluate it rationally and respond with affirmations of what's good about yourself.

Here are some examples:

Negative or irrational beliefs	Positive or rational beliefs
Because of my pain, I'm no longer the person I was. I'm no longer loved and appreciated.	I'm worthy of love, and I'm worthy of being appreciated for all that I am.
People reject me because they can see I'm disabled.	I'm not disabled. I have goals, dreams and I can do many things.
I can't do all that I used to. I'm no longer competent or adequate.	I can do much of what I want to. As long as I don't overdo, I can be actively involved in life.
I have no control over my happiness. Pain controls me.	I can control my happiness. I can enjoy life regardless of pain.
I used to be able to do so many things. Now I can't do anything.	I can do a lot more than I thought. Almost everything I used to do I can still do to some degree.
If I go out with friends and my pain acts up, I won't be able to manage. I'll embarrass myself and ruin things for everyone.	I can enjoy friends and have a good time. I may take breaks from my usual activities, but it can still be fun.
People at work are upset with me. They think I'm not doing my share of the work.	I will do the best job I can. My co-workers will have to learn to accept my limitations.
Medical science can do so much. Certainly there must be a cure for my pain.	Medical science can't fix everything. Many medical problems aren't cured but controlled.

Types of distorted thinking

Here are some common forms of negative, irrational thinking. Try to identify and challenge these thoughts:

Filtering. You magnify the negative aspects of a situation and filter out all of the positive ones. For example, you had a great day at work. You completed your tasks ahead of time and were complimented for your speedy and thorough work. But you forgot one minor step. That evening you focus only on your oversight and forget about the compliments paid you.

Personalizing. When something bad occurs, you automatically think that you're to blame. For example, you hear that a family picnic has been canceled, and you start thinking the change in plans is because no one wanted to be around you.

Generalizing. You see a troubling event as the beginning of an unending cycle. When your pain failed to go away, your thoughts may have followed this path: "I'll never be able to do what I used to. I'm a burden to everyone around me. I'm worthless."

Catastrophizing. You automatically anticipate the worst. You refuse to go out with friends for fear your pain will act up and you'll make a fool of yourself. Or one change in your daily routine leads you to think the day will be a disaster.

Polarizing. You see things only as black and white, good or bad. There's no middle ground. You feel you have to be perfect or you're a failure.

Emotionalizing. With this type of distorted thinking you allow your feelings to control your judgment. If you feel stupid and boring, then you must be stupid and boring.

Challenging your expectations

Some people are perfectionists, constantly striving for excellence. These are the homemakers whose house could pass a military white-glove inspection, the master welders who pride themselves on their precision work and the grandparents who never miss their grandchild's soccer games.

This compulsive perfectionism isn't the lifestyle for someone with chronic pain. Trying to live up to a perfectionist's expectations can become emotionally and physically damaging.

Before pain invaded your life, perhaps you could work 50 to 60 hours a week with no problem, clean your entire house in 2 hours and play a set of tennis every Saturday. Now, even part-time work leaves you exhausted, household chores become intimidating day-long projects and tennis is unimaginable.

As long as you compare yourself with how you used to be, you'll feel miserable about your performance. Your work won't be good enough, and your leisure time won't be enjoyable enough.

There is, however, a way to keep an upbeat outlook, and that's to become a perfectionist at adjusting your goals. People who don't adapt to new challenges are more likely to become discouraged and depressed. But those who are flexible enough to adjust their expectations generally have a positive attitude about life and manage to stay active. "I can't work a full-time job and still keep a perfect house," you might say to yourself, "but I can at least clean up the dirty dishes in the kitchen and make sure the floors aren't littered with newspapers and clothes."

Whatever new projects you take on or goals you set for yourself, don't focus only on the outcome. Learn to enjoy the process, not just the completion of the task. Look at it as an opportunity to learn and grow.

Learning to assert yourself

Responding to all of the challenges of daily life can be difficult. And sometimes, one of the toughest tasks is learning to say no, even when doing so is in your best interest. To keep from disappointing others, you do things you know you shouldn't. You spend all day on your feet shopping with a friend. You agree to stay late at work to finish a last-minute project. This is passive behavior. You put your thoughts, feelings and health aside for the sake of others. Passive behavior can stem from your upbringing and your beliefs about the importance of helping others and treating them with respect. Or it can result from low self-esteem.

Unfortunately, passive behavior and chronic pain can be a dangerous combination. When you continually give in to the wishes of others — at your expense — your frustration can grow, your self-esteem erode and your pain increase.

Aggressive behavior isn't any better. Contrary to passive behavior, aggressive behavior is being insensitive to others or accomplishing your goals at their expense. Examples include voicing your opinions in such a way that you intimidate others from speaking up or barging ahead of people who are waiting patiently. This type of behavior can lower your self-respect, alienate relationships and leave you lonely.

Passive-aggressive behavior is also self-defeating. Getting even instead of expressing anger directly leads to more conflict. Giving someone the silent treatment or being intentionally late for an appointment can lead to further stress in your relationship which, in turn, can contribute to physical tension and increased pain. So, how do you stand up for yourself without being blunt or hurtful to others? The answer is assertive behavior. Assertive behavior is honestly and openly expressing your feelings while at the same time showing concern for the feelings of others.

Here's an example. "I miss spending time with all of you, and I'd like to go golfing with the group. But instead of playing 18 holes, I'm going to bow out after 9 and wait for you to finish. I hope you can understand."

Assertive behavior is based on *I* statements. (The word *I* is used four times in the previous paragraph.) *I* statements allow you to tell people exactly how you feel and what you think, without placing blame or creating feelings of guilt.

Steps to being more assertive

These suggestions can help you be more assertive when communicating with others:

Observe your behavior. Honestly evaluate your behavior when speaking with others. Are there times when you're assertive, such as when communicating with a certain co-worker or family member, or are you always passive or aggressive?

Make a mental note of situations in which you responded well and those in which you feel you could have done better.

Think before you respond. When you want to make a statement or you're asked a question, think briefly about the best way to get your point across assertively, instead of simply blurting out an automatic response.

Plan for a difficult situation. Think about a situation you're likely to encounter in which you'll need to be assertive. Close your eyes and imagine how you'll respond. What might the person say? What will you say in return?

Here's an example. Your company is making plans to launch a new product, and you know your boss is going to ask you to head up the launch committee because you can never say no. But you're having trouble keeping up with your duties as it is, and you know the stress and long days involved to get the product ready would be difficult.

Picture your boss walking into your office and sitting in the chair by your desk. When your boss says, "I'd really like you to take on this assignment," practice your response: "I understand the importance of this project. However, my schedule is already very full, and I need to keep from overextending myself. If there's another way I can help that doesn't require as much time, I'm happy to do it." In addition, repeating statements may be necessary as you change to a more assertive communication style.

Pay attention to your body language. As you practice being more assertive, observe how you stand or sit, along with your gestures, facial expressions and eye contact. For example, when talking to someone, do you look at the person? Or do you stare at the ceiling or floor or out a window?

Boosting your self-esteem

Your struggle with chronic pain can result in some damaging blows to your self-image. Some of these are self-imposed, such as your inability to measure up to your own expectations. Others may come from family, friends, colleagues or even strangers. Perhaps they criticize or ignore you because you don't meet their standards or because you look haggard from your struggle with pain.

It's important to maintain a strong sense of self-worth. The better you feel about yourself, the better you'll take care of yourself.

In addition, a positive self-image has been linked to a stronger immune system. Feeling good about yourself may actually improve your health.

Many of the steps discussed in this chapter — managing your anger, practicing positive thinking, challenging your expectations and learning to assert yourself — will have a positive effect on your self-esteem. As you learn how to control and express your emotions, you'll feel better about yourself and more confident in your abilities, and your self-image will improve.

There may be days, however, when your self-esteem could use a little energizing. When that happens, consider these suggestions:

Structure your day with goals you can meet. When the day is done, you'll feel a sense of accomplishment.

Talk with a friend. Having someone who's willing to take time to listen lets you know that you're valued.

Spend time with others. It will make you feel more connected and less alone.

Help someone. It reminds you that your life makes a difference.

Treat yourself to something you enjoy. This might be some new music, a great book or a scoop of your favorite ice cream. Just as you buy gifts for others who are feeling down, you need to do the same for yourself.

Spruce up your appearance. Try a different hairstyle. Buy some new clothes. The better you look, the better you feel about yourself.

List reasons people like you. It reminds you that you have special qualities people enjoy.

List things you do well. Then do one of them.

Chapter 13

Managing stress

Pain and stress go hand in hand. When you're in pain, you're less able to handle the stress of everyday life. Common hassles turn into major obstacles. Stress may also cause you to do things that intensify your pain, such as tense your muscles, grit your teeth and stiffen your shoulders. In short, pain causes stress, and stress intensifies pain.

The first step in breaking this pain-stress cycle is to realize that stress is your response to an event, not the event itself. It's something you can control. That's why events that are stressful for some people aren't for others. For example, your morning commute may leave you anxious and tense because you use it as worry time. Your co-worker, however, finds her commute relaxing. She enjoys her time alone without distractions. Understanding that you have control over your stress can help you develop positive strategies for dealing with stress.

How you respond to stress

When you encounter stress, your body responds in a manner similar to a physical threat. It automatically gears up to face the challenge or musters the strength necessary to get out of trouble's way.

This fight-or-flight response results from the release of hormones that cause your body to shift into overdrive. Your heart beats faster, your blood pressure increases and your breathing quickens and becomes more shallow. Your nervous system also springs into action, causing your facial muscles to tighten and your body to perspire more.

Stress can be negative or positive:

- Positive stress provides a feeling of excitement and opportunity. Positive stress often helps athletes perform better in competition than in practice. Other examples of positive stress include a new job or birth of a child.
- Negative stress occurs when you feel out of control or under constant or intense pressure. You may have trouble concentrating, or you may feel alone. Family, finances, work, isolation and health problems, including pain, are common causes of negative stress.

Continued stress can have a negative effect on your health. In addition to the strain it puts on your cardiovascular system, the hormone cortisol released during stress may suppress your immune system, making you more susceptible to infections and disease. Stress can also cause headaches and worsen intestinal problems and asthma.

What are your triggers?

Stress is often associated with situations or events that you find difficult to handle. How you view things also affects your level of stress. If you have unrealistic or high expectations, chances are you'll experience more than your fair share of stress.

Take some time to think about what causes you stress. Your stress may be linked to external factors, such as:

- Community
- Environment
- Family
- Unpredictable events
- Work

Stress can also come from internal factors, such as:

- Irresponsible behavior
- Negative attitudes and feelings
- Perfectionism
- Poor health habits
- Unrealistic expectations

Jot down what seem to be sources of stress for you. And then ask yourself if there's anything you can do to lessen or avoid them. There are some stressors you can control and some you can't.

Concentrate on events you can change. For situations that are beyond your control, look for ways to adapt — to remain calm under trying circumstances.

Strategies for reducing stress

It's one thing to be aware of stress in your daily life, but it's another to know how to change it. As you look through your list of stressors, think carefully about why they're so bothersome. For example, if your busy day is a source of stress, ask yourself if it's because you tend to squeeze too many things into your day or because you aren't organized.

The following techniques can help you reduce those sources of stress you can control and better cope with those you can't.

Change your lifestyle

Consider these changes to your normal routine:

Plan your day. This can help you feel more in control of your life. You might start by getting up 15 minutes earlier to ease the morning rush. Do unpleasant tasks early in the day and be done with them. Keep a written schedule of your daily activities so that you're not faced with conflicts or last-minute rushes (see "Your personal planner" on page 181). Because a pain flare-up can happen at any time, have a backup plan — decide what you can do now and what can wait.

Simplify your schedule. Prioritize, plan and pace yourself. Learn to delegate responsibility to others at home and at work. Say no to added responsibilities or commitments if you're not up to doing them. And try not to feel guilty if you aren't productive every waking moment.

Get organized. Organize your home and work space so that you know where things are. Keep your house, car and personal belongings in working order to prevent untimely and stressful repairs.

Take breaks. Take time to relax, stretch or walk periodically during the day.

Exercise regularly. Regular physical activity helps loosen your muscles and relieves emotional intensity. Try to exercise for a total of at least 30 minutes most days of the week.

Get enough sleep. This can give you the energy you need to face each day. Going to sleep and awakening at a consistent time also may help you sleep more soundly.

Eat well. A diet that includes a variety of foods provides the right mix of nutrients to keep your body systems working well. When you're healthy, you're better able to control stress and pain.

Change the pace. Occasionally break away from your routine and explore new territory without a schedule. Take a vacation, even if it's just a weekend getaway.

Be positive. There's no room for "Yes, but .... " Avoiding negative self-talk can be difficult. It helps to spend time with people who have a positive outlook and a sense of humor. Laughter actually helps ease pain. It releases endorphins, chemicals in your brain that give you a sense of well-being.

Stay connected. Recognize when you need the support of family and friends. Talking about your problems with others can often relieve pent-up emotions and lead to solutions you hadn't thought of on your own.

Be patient. Realizing that improvements in your health may take time can help reduce anxiety and stress.

Relief through relaxation

You can't avert all sources of stress, such as an unexpected visit from family or friends or a problem at work. However, you can modify how you react to these situations by practicing relaxation techniques. Relaxation helps relieve stress that can aggravate chronic pain. It also helps prevent muscle spasms and reduces muscle tension.

Relaxation won't cure your pain, but it can:
- Reduce anxiety and conserve energy
- Increase your self-control when dealing with stress
- Help you recognize the difference between tense muscles and relaxed ones

- Help you physically and emotionally handle your daily demands
- Help you remain alert, energetic and productive

Keep in mind, though, that the benefits of relaxation are only as good as your efforts. Learning to relax takes time.

Techniques to try

There are many ways to relax, so pick one that works best for you.

Deep breathing. Unlike children, most adults breathe from their chest. Each time you breathe in, your chest expands, and each time you breathe out, it contracts. Children, however, generally breathe from their diaphragm, the muscle that separates the chest from the abdomen. Deep breathing from your diaphragm — which adults can relearn — is relaxing. It also exchanges more carbon dioxide for oxygen, to give you more energy. Try to incorporate 20 minutes of deep breathing every day for good health, not just when you're stressed (see "Taking a breather" on page 148).

Progressive muscle relaxation. This technique involves relaxing a series of muscles one at a time. First, raise the tension level in a group of muscles, such as in a leg or an arm, by tightening the muscles and then relaxing them. Concentrate on letting the tension go in each muscle. Then move on to the next muscle group. Be careful, however, not to tense muscles near your pain sites.

Word repetition. Choose a word or phrase that is a cue for you to relax, and then repeat it. While repeating the word or phrase, try to breathe deeply and slowly and think of something that gives you pleasant sensations of warmth and heaviness.

Guided imagery. Also known as visualization, this method of relaxation involves lying quietly and picturing yourself in a pleasant and peaceful setting. You experience the setting with all of your senses as if you were actually there. For instance, imagine lying on the beach. Picture the beautiful blue sky, smell the salt water, hear the waves and feel the warm breeze on your skin. The messages your brain receives as you experience these senses help you to relax.

Taking a breather

Here's an exercise to help you practice deep, relaxed diaphragmatic breathing. Practice it throughout the day until it becomes natural so that you can use it readily when you feel stressed.

- Lie down on your back or sit comfortably with your feet flat on the floor.
- Rest one hand on your abdomen and one hand on your chest.
- Inhale through your nose while pushing your abdomen out.
- Slowly exhale through your nose while gently relaxing your abdomen. Make each breath a smooth, wave-like motion.
- If you have difficulty breathing through your nose, breathe through your mouth.
- Take normal, not deep breaths. Practicing this way will make it easier to use in stressful situations.

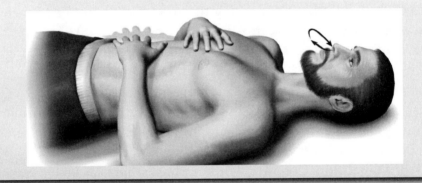

Tips to help you succeed

Practice. If relaxation is new to you, you may not notice immediate benefits. In fact, you may feel uncomfortable at first. Work on your relaxation skills at least once or twice a day until they come naturally. When you're beginning, a quiet place and a relaxation tape often help.

Get comfortable. Loosen tight clothing and remove your shoes and belt, if need be.

Vary your schedule. Practice relaxation at different times throughout the day. The idea is to learn how to relax whenever you need to.

Be patient. A wandering mind is normal when you start out. Just keep bringing your attention back to relaxation.

Chapter 14

Interacting with family and friends

As trying as your chronic pain is for you, it can be every bit as troubling to your family and friends. They want to help you, but they may not know how. So they say or do things they think are helpful but may only add to your frustration.

Because chronic pain is such a personal experience, it's difficult for family and friends to understand exactly what you're going through. In addition, when pain takes over, communication often suffers. You may not feel like discussing your pain or the problems related to it. And family and friends may hesitate to approach certain topics for fear they'll anger or frustrate you.

You need family and friends to help you manage your pain and move on with your life. But your family and friends can help you only if you help them.

Benefits of social interaction

People with a solid support system have many health advantages. For example, people with caring family and friends generally:
- Cope better with chronic pain
- Are less likely to experience depression
- Are more independent
- Recover faster from illness
- Live longer

Through your own experiences, you may know what researchers are talking about. You've felt how quickly a cup of coffee with a neighbor has lifted your spirits. You've experienced how a helping hand from a relative has helped you get through a bad day. And you know how even a short trip with a friend can invigorate you. Being around others can help you forget about your frustrations.

Developing a strong support system

Good friends and a supportive family can provide encouraging words, offer gentle but helpful criticisms and lend a hand when you need assistance. Family and friends also help replace sadness with smiles and laughter. In this way, they contribute to your health and well-being.

Making friendships and maintaining family ties seem to come more naturally for some people than for others. But even if you're not an outgoing person, you need social support. If your support system is in need of a little strengthening, try these suggestions:

- Answer phone calls and letters.
- Accept invitations to events, even if it feels awkward and difficult at first.
- Don't wait to be invited somewhere. Take the initiative and call someone.
- Set aside past differences and approach your relationships with a clean slate.
- Take part in community organizations, neighborhood events and family gatherings.
- Strike up a conversation with the person next to you at a local gathering. You could be introducing yourself to a new friend.
- Talk about things that other people are interested in. And be an alert listener.

Good relationships require patience, compromise and acceptance. Without these things, the relationship can become a source of stress instead of support. Family and friends need to learn to accept you along with your needs, and you need to accept them along with theirs.

It's true that relationships can sometimes be difficult. Your friends and family may want more of your time and energy than

How does your social network stack up?

A strong support system is associated with better health and a longer life. Check each statement that's true about your relationships. Each statement marks an important link in your social network.

_____ I have friends or family members nearby to help me.

_____ I'm involved in a community or religious organization.

_____ I have at least one friend or relative that I can talk to about almost anything.

_____ I keep in daily contact with other people.

Statements you didn't mark are areas you might work on to improve your support system.

you can spare. But instead of drawing away from those you're close to, educate them about your pain. And allow friends and family members to tell you how your pain has affected them.

This will help those closest to you understand why you may not always be able to keep up with them or do all of the things they ask. It will also help you understand how your pain affects others.

Improving your communication skills

Discussing your thoughts and feelings can be difficult even in the best of times. With chronic pain, the task doesn't get any easier. Instead of continually telling people what you're going through and how you're feeling, it's often easier to withdraw or say as little as possible.

The problem with this approach, however, is that it can frustrate and alienate your family and friends. They may not know how to interpret your withdrawal and won't know that you're having a bad day unless you tell them. You don't have to go on about your symptoms, but simply saying "I'm having a rough day" or "I need some space" will let them know you need time to yourself.

So how do you improve communication?

Express what you're feeling. The only way people can begin to understand what you're thinking or feeling is if you tell them. But do it in a positive manner, not one in which you appear to be whining or accusatory. Negative emotions only increase your chances for a negative response.

For example, if you're frustrated because your friends don't include you in their activities anymore, you might say, "I miss spending time with you on Saturdays, and I sure would like to join you on a walk or bicycling." Your friends may incorrectly assume that you can't take part in recreational events. That's why they don't invite you to join them, not because they don't want to be around you.

Don't lie about your pain. Close family and friends may know not to ask how you're doing every time they see you. But some people won't understand that you may always have some degree of pain. When they inquire how you're doing, don't pretend it doesn't hurt. But don't exaggerate your pain, either. You might respond, "I still have pain, but I'm learning to manage it."

Ask for help when you need it. You were probably taught to cherish your independence, so it may be difficult for you to ask for help. But sometimes you need help. Try asking in a way that explains what's going on. For example: "I've invited friends over for dinner, and it's taking me longer to get the meal prepared than I anticipated. I look forward to having friends come, but I need some help. Could you please come over and lend me a hand for a while?"

Be a cheerful receiver. When someone helps you or gives you a heartfelt compliment about your progress, say thanks. Try not to feel depressed that you needed the help or the emotional boost.

Discuss communication roadblocks. If the flow of communication between you and a family member or friend becomes one-sided, talk about it. Set aside your pride for a while and take the risk of saying exactly how you feel. If that fails to open the channel, don't give up too soon. Consider asking advice from a counselor.

Put your toughest communication problems in writing. Use your journal to express those feelings you have trouble communicating. This not only will buy you some time to let these feelings settle but also will give you practice in expressing them when you're ready to discuss them.

Ways family and friends can help

Chances are your family and friends have asked you what they can do to help you. Perhaps you didn't know what to say, or you felt guilty admitting that you needed any type of special treatment. Or maybe they've decided to help in ways that irritate you. They think they're doing things to make you feel better, but they're not.

When people ask you how they can help, tell them. Here are some suggestions you might pass along:

Learn more about my pain. Chronic pain is difficult to understand. Reading about it will help family and friends better understand what you're going through, how they can help and when they shouldn't help. For instance, continually doing tasks for you that you can do for yourself unintentionally contributes to your loss of independence and self-confidence.

Don't let conversations always gravitate to my pain. It's easy for friends and family to get caught up in discussing your pain. But that only reminds you of your condition and draws attention to your pain — something you're trying to avoid.

Try not to hover over me. Being overly attentive to someone with persistent pain can actually interfere with rehabilitation. One study found that people with chronic pain who were observed by an overly attentive spouse reported more pain than when they were observed by someone else.

Tell your spouse or partner that you appreciate the concern, but that he or she doesn't need to be your servant. To manage your pain, you need to learn to do things for yourself. Many studies confirm that when family members, in particular, are supportive in upbeat and positive ways that don't reinforce pain behaviors, such as limping, groaning or grimacing, the person with chronic pain has a much better prognosis.

Join me in activities. Having friends and family members accompany you for a walk or go with you to support meetings or doctor visits can offer many benefits. Having friends or family members along gives you a chance to talk and share time together. It also gives friends and family members an opportunity to learn more about your need to exercise and stay active.

Don't give up things you enjoy for my sake. Those closest to you may consciously or unconsciously change their lifestyle because of your pain. But that doesn't encourage you, and it may make you feel guilty. For example, if you and a friend enjoyed fishing together, don't let your friend sell his tackle just because he thinks you can't fish anymore. Perhaps you can't fish from dawn to dusk as you used to, but you may be able to fish for a few hours.

Be available to listen to me. Sometimes you simply need someone to listen. A family member or friend who understands that you're not asking them to fix the problem can lend emotional support by just listening to you. This often provides a release valve for your daily stresses. People with chronic pain who feel they have the support of loved ones seem to cope better with their pain, return to work sooner and live more active lives.

As they listen, your family members and friends can help you by reminding you of the progress you're making and keeping you focused on positive solutions to your problems.

Take care of yourself. Your pain, and worrying about you, can take a toll on friends and family members. It's important that those you care about take care of their health as well. Just as you need their support, they need yours.

Chapter 15

Caring for yourself

L iving well with chronic pain isn't just about managing your pain. It's about caring for your overall health so that you can enjoy life to its fullest.

Improving physical fitness, reducing stress and learning to relax have all been covered in earlier chapters. Now it's time to focus on other factors that can help you stay active and productive and feel good about yourself.

Getting a good night's sleep

Sleep refreshes you. It improves your attitude and gives you energy for physical activity and to fight off fatigue and stress. It also boosts your immune system, reducing your risk of illness.

If you aren't sleeping well, it may be because your pain is keeping you from falling asleep or is waking you up at night. Other factors that can interfere with sleep are:

- Stress
- Anxiety
- Depression
- Alcohol
- Poor sleep habits
- Stimulant medications
- Regular use of over-the-counter sleeping pills
- Lack of physical activity
- Change in your environment

To improve your sleep, it's important to recognize factors that may be contributing to your restless nights.

Stages of sleep

There are two types of sleep — rapid eye movement (REM) and nonrapid eye movement (NREM). As you pass from being awake to being asleep (transitional sleep) you're in stage 1 of NREM sleep. There are three other stages of NREM sleep. Stage 2 is the most frequent stage. Stages 3 and 4, which are called delta sleep, are the most restful. During NREM sleep, your brain activity and body functions slow.

REM sleep is a period of increased activity. This is the phase of sleep during which you dream and your body functions speed up. Early REM periods are very short, usually 5 to 10 minutes in length. REM periods during the second part of the night are longer, usually lasting about 20 to 40 minutes. Because REM sleep is active sleep, people often feel that sleep during the second half of the night is much shallower than the first half.

Throughout the night, you continually move from one stage or type of sleep to another in cycles that can last from 70 to 90 minutes each.

NREM is the most restful kind of sleep. It's also the type of sleep that many people with chronic pain miss. If you have trouble falling asleep, frequently awaken at night or wake up feeling as though you haven't slept at all, you may not be reaching periods of NREM sleep. Instead, you spend your night in REM sleep. And though REM sleep helps refresh your body, it doesn't provide the relaxation and energy boost you receive from NREM sleep.

Strategies to help you sleep better

Before bed, take time to relax. That might include:

- Practicing relaxation techniques
- Having a light snack
- Listening to soothing music
- Taking a warm bath
- Reading
- Writing in your journal

Relaxation helps reduce your pain so that you can fall asleep more easily. It also helps you achieve more restful sleep.

Here are other suggestions that may help you sleep better:

Establish regular sleep hours. Go to bed and wake up at the same time each day. Following a regular pattern often improves sleep.

Limit your time in bed. Too much sleep can promote shallow, unrestful sleep. Contrary to expectations, spending too much time in bed usually disrupts sleep in the middle of the night. Nine out of 10 people with insomnia stay in bed longer than necessary.

Don't try to sleep. The harder you try, the more awake you'll become. Read or watch television until you become drowsy and fall asleep naturally.

Limit bedroom activities. Save your bedroom for sleep and sex. Don't watch TV or take your work materials to bed.

Watch what you eat. A light snack may help you relax before sleeping. However, avoid heavy meals and fluids or foods that stimulate stomach acid production, which could cause heartburn or irritate your esophagus (esophageal reflux).

Avoid or limit caffeine, alcohol and nicotine. Caffeine and nicotine can keep you from falling asleep. Alcohol can cause unrestful sleep and frequent awakening.

Minimize interruptions. Close your bedroom door or create a subtle background noise, such as that from a fan, to muffle other noises. Drink less before bed so that you won't have to get up at night to go to the bathroom.

Get comfy. Make sure you have a bed that's comfortable and keep your bedroom temperature at a comfortably cool level.

Hide the clock. A visible readout of how long you've been unable to sleep may make you needlessly anxious. Place clocks where they aren't visible or within reach so that you won't keep checking the time.

Keep active. Regular physical activity helps you sleep more soundly. Try to get at least 30 minutes of physical activity daily, preferably 5 to 6 hours before bedtime. Also keep occupied throughout the day. Boredom promotes restless sleep.

Avoid or limit naps. Naps can make it harder to fall asleep at night. (See "To nap, or not?")

Schedule worry time. Don't take your worries to bed with you. During the evening, address your worries and ways to solve them.

To nap, or not?

The urge for a midday snooze is built into your body's biological clock. It generally occurs between 1 p.m. and 4 p.m., when your body temperature naturally dips slightly.

Napping isn't a substitute for a full night's sleep. Don't nap if you have trouble sleeping at night. If you find a nap refreshes you and doesn't interfere with nighttime sleep, try these ideas:

Keep it short. Thirty minutes is ideal. Naps longer than 1 to 2 hours are more likely to interfere with your nighttime sleep.

Take a midafternoon nap. Naps at this time produce a physically invigorating slumber.

If you can't nap, just rest. Lie down and keep your mind on something relaxing.

Check your medications. Ask your doctor if they might be contributing to your difficulty sleeping. Also check over-the-counter products that you're taking to see if they contain caffeine or other stimulants, such as pseudoephedrine.

What about sleep medications?

If you're having trouble sleeping, your doctor may prescribe a medication until other steps to improve your sleep and control your pain have time to take effect. The downfall of many prescription and over-the-counter sleep medications is that they often don't allow you to experience all phases of sleep. The drugs can also lose their effectiveness and cause side effects, including dry mouth, next-day drowsiness and physical dependence. That's why it's best to try to improve your sleep with changes in your lifestyle.

For sleep difficulties associated with chronic pain, antidepressants are often prescribed. A side effect of some antidepressants is drowsiness. When taken before bed, they can help you sleep. Plus, antidepressants aren't addictive.

Controlling your weight

Maintaining a healthy weight reduces your risk of illnesses such as cardiovascular disease, high blood pressure and diabetes. It's also easier to manage your pain when you're not overweight. That's because excessive weight saps your energy level, increases stress on muscles and joints and decreases your flexibility. It's not necessary that you become thin. But losing even a few pounds may help reduce your level of pain, as well as your blood sugar and cholesterol levels.

Is your weight healthy?

Three do-it-yourself evaluations can tell you if your weight is healthy or whether you could benefit from weight loss.

Body mass index. Body mass index (BMI) is a formula that considers your weight and your height in determining whether you have a healthy or unhealthy percentage of total body fat. It's a better measurement of health risks related to your weight than using your bathroom scale or standard height and weight tables.

To determine your BMI, locate your height on the chart ("What's your BMI?") on the next page and follow it across until you reach the weight nearest yours. Look at the top of the column for the BMI rating. If your weight is less than the weight nearest yours, your BMI may be slightly less. If your weight is greater than the weight nearest yours, your BMI may be slightly greater. A BMI of 18.5 to 24.9 is considered healthy. A BMI of 25.0 to 29.9 signifies overweight, and a BMI of 30 or more indicates obesity.

Waist circumference. This measurement indicates where most of your body fat is located. People who carry most of their weight around their waists may be referred to as apple-like. Those who carry most of their weight below their waists, around their hips and thighs, may be described as pear-like.

Generally, it's better to have a pear shape than an apple shape. That's because fat around your abdomen is associated with a greater risk of cardiovascular and other weight-related diseases.

To determine whether you're carrying too much weight around your abdomen, measure your waist circumference. Find the

What's your BMI?

Body mass index (BMI)

BMI	Healthy		Overweight					Obesity				
	19	**24**	25	26	27	28	29	30	35	40	45	50
Height					Weight in pounds							
4'10"	91	115	119	124	129	134	138	143	167	191	215	239
4'11"	94	119	124	128	133	138	143	148	173	198	222	247
5'0"	97	123	128	133	138	143	148	153	179	204	230	255
5'1"	100	127	132	137	143	148	153	158	185	211	238	264
5'2"	104	131	136	142	147	153	158	164	191	218	246	273
5'3"	107	135	141	146	152	158	163	169	197	225	254	282
5'4"	110	140	145	151	157	163	169	174	204	232	262	291
5'5"	114	144	150	156	162	168	174	180	210	240	270	300
5'6"	118	148	155	161	167	173	179	186	216	247	278	309
5'7"	121	153	159	166	172	178	185	191	223	255	287	319
5'8"	125	158	164	171	177	184	190	197	230	262	295	328
5'9"	128	162	169	176	182	189	196	203	236	270	304	338
5'10"	132	167	174	181	188	195	202	209	243	278	313	348
5'11"	136	172	179	186	193	200	208	215	250	286	322	358
6'0"	140	177	184	191	199	206	213	221	258	294	331	368
6'1"	144	182	189	197	204	212	219	227	265	302	340	378
6'2"	148	186	194	202	210	218	225	233	272	311	350	389
6'3"	152	192	200	208	216	224	232	240	279	319	359	399
6'4"	156	197	205	213	221	230	238	246	287	328	369	410

Adapted from National Institutes of Health *Clinical Guidelines on the Identification, Evaluation, and Treatment of Overweight and Obesity in Adults,* 1998.

highest point on each of your hipbones and measure across your abdomen just above those points. A measurement of more than 40 inches (102 centimeters) in men and 35 inches (89 centimeters) in women signifies increased health risks, especially if you have a BMI of 25 or more.

Personal and family history. An evaluation of your medical history, along with that of your family, is equally important in determining whether your weight is healthy.

Answer these questions:

- Do you have a health condition, such as arthritis or back pain, that would benefit from weight loss?
- Do you have a family history of a weight-related illness, such as diabetes, high blood pressure or high cholesterol?
- Have you gained considerable weight since high school? Weight gain in adulthood is associated with increased health risks.
- Do you smoke cigarettes, have more than two alcoholic drinks a day or live with considerable stress? In combination with these behaviors, excess weight can have greater health implications.

Adding up the results. If your BMI shows you aren't overweight, you're not carrying too much weight around your abdomen and you answered no to all of the personal or family history questions, there's probably no health advantage to changing your weight. Your weight is healthy.

If your BMI is between 25.0 and 29.9, your waist circumference exceeds healthy guidelines or you answered yes to at least one personal and family health question, you might benefit from losing a few pounds. Discuss your weight with your doctor during your next visit.

If your BMI is 30 or more, losing weight will improve your overall health and energy level and reduce your risk of future illness.

Losing weight successfully

The best way to lose weight safely and keep it off permanently is through lifestyle changes. There are many products and programs that promise to help you shed pounds, but they aren't always safe or effective. Once you go off the diet, you gain the weight back again.

Here are some steps that can help you be successful:

Make a commitment. You must be motivated to lose weight because it's what you want, not what someone else wants you to do. Only you can lose weight. However, that doesn't mean that you have to do everything alone. Your doctor or a registered dietitian can help you plan how best to lose weight.

Think positively. Don't dwell on what you're giving up to lose weight. Instead, concentrate on what you're gaining. Instead of thinking, "I really miss eating a doughnut for breakfast," tell yourself, "I feel a lot better when I eat whole-wheat toast and cereal in the morning."

Set a realistic goal. Don't aim for a weight that's unrealistic. If you've always been overweight, aim for a weight that will help reduce pressure on your joints and muscles and improve your energy level. Studies show that losing even 10 percent of what you weigh can improve your health and sense of well-being.

Accept that healthy weight loss is slow and steady. A good weight loss plan generally involves losing no more than 1 to 2 pounds (0.5 to 1 kilogram) a week. Set weekly or monthly goals that allow you to check off your successes. Reward yourself when you meet a goal.

Know your habits. Ask yourself if you tend to eat when you're bored, angry, tired, anxious, depressed or socially pressured. If you do, try these possible solutions:

- Before eating anything, ask yourself if you really want it.
- Do something to distract yourself from your desire to eat, such as telephone a friend or run an errand.
- If you're feeling stressed or angry, direct that energy constructively. Instead of eating, practice a relaxation technique or take a brisk walk.

Don't starve yourself. Liquid meals, diet pills and special food combinations aren't your answer to long-term weight control and better health.

Most people try to lose weight by eating 1,000 to 1,500 calories a day. Cutting calories to fewer than 1,200 if you're a woman or 1,400 if you're a man doesn't provide enough food to keep you satisfied.

Plus it promotes temporary loss of fluids and loss of healthy muscle, instead of permanent loss of fat.

The best way to lose weight is through healthy eating.

Get and stay active. Dieting alone will help you lose weight. But by adding 30 minutes of moderate activity most days of the week, you can increase your rate of weight loss.

Only you will know how much you can exercise. Pain may impose limits on the types of exercise you do. However, exercise may also relieve pain and stiffness.

Physical activity is the most important factor related to long-term weight loss. It promotes loss of body fat and development of muscle. These changes in body composition help raise the rate at which you burn calories, making it easier to maintain your weight loss.

Think lifelong. It's not enough to eat healthy foods and exercise for a few weeks or even several months. As with other strategies for managing your pain, you have to incorporate these new behaviors into your life.

Eating for better health

Food can't control your pain. But a nutritionally balanced diet can improve the way you feel. In addition to helping you lose weight, eating a variety of foods gives you energy and a sense of well-being. Nutritious foods, combined with a healthy weight, are also your best bet for staying healthy.

Experts agree that the best way to increase nutrients in your diet and limit fat and calories is to eat more plant-based foods. Plant foods — fruits, vegetables and foods made from whole grains — contain beneficial vitamins, minerals, fibers and health-enhancing compounds called phytochemicals. By emphasizing plant foods in your diet, you increase consumption of many naturally healthy compounds.

For good health and better success at controlling your weight, here are the types and amounts of foods to eat each day. The recommendations are based on the Mayo Clinic Healthy Weight Pyramid — a healthy eating plan for all Americans.

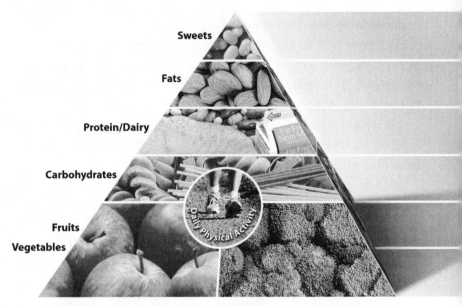

Sweets

Fats

Protein/Dairy

Carbohydrates

Fruits

Vegetables

Mayo Clinic Healthy Weight Pyramid

Vegetables: Unlimited servings. Vegetables are naturally low in calories, and almost all are fat-free. They provide vitamins, minerals and fiber. They also contain phytochemicals.

Fresh vegetables are best, but frozen vegetables are good, too. Most canned vegetables are high in sodium, which is used as a preservative in the canning process. Excessive sodium can increase blood pressure in some people. If you eat canned vegetables, select those with a label indicating that no sodium has been added.

Fruits: Unlimited servings. Fruit is generally low in calories and contains little or no fat. Fruit also contains many beneficial nutrients and phytochemicals.

Fresh fruit is always best. It makes a great snack. If you get the urge to snack between meals or you have a sweet tooth, keep a bowl of fresh fruit nearby. Frozen fruits with no added sugar and fruits canned in water or their own juices are acceptable alternatives. Eat dried fruits, such as dates and prunes, sparingly because they're a concentrated source of calories. Fruit juice also is a concentrated source of calories. Avocados contain considerable calories and fat, and their consumption should be limited.

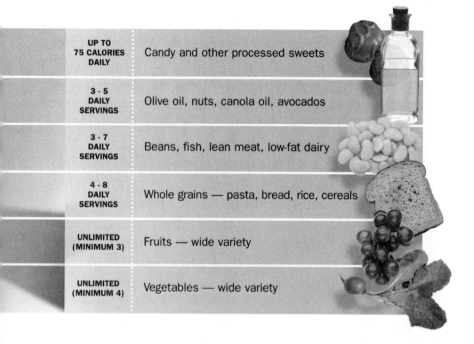

UP TO 75 CALORIES DAILY	Candy and other processed sweets
3 - 5 DAILY SERVINGS	Olive oil, nuts, canola oil, avocados
3 - 7 DAILY SERVINGS	Beans, fish, lean meat, low-fat dairy
4 - 8 DAILY SERVINGS	Whole grains — pasta, bread, rice, cereals
UNLIMITED (MINIMUM 3)	Fruits — wide variety
UNLIMITED (MINIMUM 4)	Vegetables — wide variety

Carbohydrates: 4 to 8 servings. Carbohydrates include grain products, such as cereals, breads, rice and pasta, and starchy vegetables, such as corn, potatoes and some types of squash.

Along with vegetables and fruits, carbohydrates should form the foundation of your daily diet. Whenever possible, select whole-grain foods over refined products. Whole grains contain bran and germ, which add fiber. Whole grains are also important sources of vitamins and minerals. Some carbohydrates, such as croissants, crackers and dessert breads, are high in fat and calories. But most plain cereals, breads and pasta are low in fat and calories. It's what you put on these foods — whole milk, cream, or spreads and sauces made from fats, oils or cheese — that adds calories.

Protein/Dairy: 3 to 7 servings. Protein is an essential nutrient that helps maintain body tissues, such as skin, bone and muscle. Protein is found in a variety of foods, including milk, yogurt, cheese, eggs, meat, poultry, fish and legumes (beans, dried peas and lentils). Most Americans eat far more protein than they need, especially those products that are high in fat and calories, such as meat.

Two to three of your daily protein servings should come from low-fat or fat-free milk or milk products (yogurt and cheese).

Milk, yogurt and cheese are major sources of calcium and vitamin D. Calcium helps keep your bones healthy and reduces your risk of osteoporosis, a disease that reduces bone density and makes your bones brittle.

Always try to select fat-free or low-fat varieties of protein, such as poultry (without skin), fish, lean meats, legumes, skim milk and low-fat cheeses.

Fats: 3 to 5 servings. A small amount of fat in your diet is necessary to help your body function, but most people consume far more than they need. Foods high in fat include products produced mainly from oils, butter, margarine, salad dressing or mayonnaise. An easy way to reduce fat in your diet is to reduce the amount of oil, butter and margarine you add to food when preparing it. Many snack products, such as chips and crackers, also are high in fat.

Healthier fats include those that contain monounsaturated fat, such as olive oil and canola oil. But even these should be eaten sparingly.

Sweets: Up to 75 calories daily. Sweets such as candy and desserts contain considerable calories, and they offer little in terms of nutrition. Many sweets are also high in fat. You don't have to give up sweets entirely to eat healthy, but be smart about your selections and portion sizes. Instead of sugar-sweetened soft drinks, candy bars or pastries, consider healthier choices, such as water, fresh fruit, low-fat frozen yogurt, angel food cake or reduced-calorie cookies.

Determining your servings for a healthy weight

The Mayo Clinic Healthy Weight Pyramid provides a range of servings for each food group. The number of servings you should eat within each range depends on a variety of factors, including your weight, activity level, age and whether you want to lose weight. If you're trying to lose weight, you'll want to aim for the lower number of servings in the food groups rather than the higher number. It's important, however, that you eat at least the minimum servings for each food group to maintain good health. A dietitian can help you determine how many servings of each food you should eat to maintain a calorie level that will help you lose weight.

As you adopt a healthier diet, it's also important to understand what constitutes a serving (see "Sizing up a serving"). With the trend toward supersizing, mega-buffets and huge portions in restaurants, many people have an inaccurate idea of what a regular portion is. Pay close attention to portion sizes. Don't just estimate. Practice at home by actually measuring and weighing cupfuls and spoonfuls.

Sizing up a serving

Here are examples of what counts as one serving:

Grains
½ cup (3 oz/90 g) cooked cereal, rice or pasta
½ cup (1 oz/30 g) ready-to-eat cereal
1 4-inch (10-cm) pancake
1 slice whole-wheat (whole-meal) sandwich bread
½ bagel or English muffin
2 cups air-popped popcorn

Vegetables and fruits
2 cups (2 oz/60 g) raw leafy green vegetables
½ cup (3 oz/90 g) cooked vegetables
1 medium potato
½ cup (3 oz/90 g) applesauce
¼ cup (1½ oz/45 g) raisins
½ cup (6 fl oz/180 mL) 100% fruit juice
1 small apple or banana

Dairy products
1 cup (8 fl oz/250 mL) low-fat or fat-free milk or yogurt
1½ oz (45 g) reduced-fat or fat-free cheese
⅔ cup (6 oz/180 g) low-fat or nonfat cottage cheese

Poultry, seafood, meat
2-3 oz (60-90 g) cooked skinless poultry, seafood or lean meat

Meat alternatives
Each of these counts as 1 oz (30 g) of meat:
  ½ cup (3½ oz/105 g) cooked legumes
  1 egg
  2 tbsp peanut butter
  ¼ cup (1 oz/30 g) seeds
  ⅓ cup (1 oz/30 g) nuts
  ½ cup (4 oz/125 g) tofu

Limiting alcohol

The best advice about alcohol is that if you drink, do it in moderation (see "What's moderate drinking?"). And if you're taking medication, it might be best not to drink any alcohol.

Alcohol can increase the potency and side effects of many prescription drugs, including pain relievers and antidepressants. In addition, regularly combining alcohol with over-the-counter pain relievers, including acetaminophen or nonsteroidal anti-inflammatory drugs, may increase your risk of liver damage.

Using alcohol to help relieve your pain can also lead to dependence and addiction. If you regularly drink more than a moderate amount of alcohol, talk with your doctor about the safest and most successful way to limit alcohol.

> ## What's moderate drinking?
>
> Moderate drinking means no more than one drink each day for women and no more than two for men. One drink equals one 12-ounce (360-milliliter, mL) bottle of beer, one 5-ounce (150-mL) glass of wine or one 1.5-ounce (45-mL) shot glass of 80-proof liquor.
>
> For men and women age 65 and older, moderate drinking is one drink daily. The amount is less for older people because they process alcohol more slowly.

Quitting smoking

There's no question smoking is dangerous to your health. Tobacco smoke contains more than 4,000 substances that can damage your heart and blood vessels and cause cancer. Smoking also contributes to chronic pain by increasing fatigue and muscle weakness. Carbon monoxide in tobacco smoke replaces oxygen in your red blood cells. Less oxygen means less energy and fewer nutrients for your body tissues.

Breaking tobacco's grip
Some people can simply stop and never smoke again. For others, quitting takes several tries and various approaches. Don't let one failed attempt to quit keep you from trying again. You can learn from previous attempts, increasing your chances for being successful in the future.

Medications to help you quit

These medications can reduce the difficult side effects of nicotine withdrawal and make quitting smoking easier. Use them according to your doctor's instructions, gradually tapering off their use over a period of weeks to months. A major advantage of these medications is that they contain no carbon monoxide or many of the 4,000 other harmful chemicals contained in tobacco smoke.

Nicotine patches. Available as over-the-counter (OTC) products and by prescription, the nicotine patch is placed on your skin, where it gradually releases nicotine into your body. This helps reduce nicotine cravings when you cut back or stop smoking. The patches can irritate your skin, but you can minimize the irritation by rotating the site of the patch.

Nicotine gum. You can also purchase OTC nicotine gum. Chew it slowly a few times, then "park" it between your cheek and gum. The lining of your mouth absorbs the nicotine the gum releases. Nicotine gum can satisfy your nicotine urge the same as the patch.

Nicotine nasal spray. It helps you quit in the same way as the patch or gum, but instead you spray nicotine into your nose. There, it's quickly absorbed into your bloodstream through the lining of your nose, providing quicker response to nicotine cravings than the other products. It's intended mainly for when you need a quick dose of nicotine and is available only by prescription.

Nicotine inhaler. The device looks like a plastic cigarette and is available only by prescription. One end of the inhaler has a plastic tip like that used on some cigars. When you put this tip in your mouth and inhale, as if puffing on a cigarette, the inhaler releases a nicotine vapor into your mouth and not your lungs, reducing your craving for nicotine.

Non-nicotine medication. Bupropion (Zyban) is the first non-nicotine medication approved by the Food and Drug Administration as a stop smoking aid. It mimics some of the action of nicotine by releasing the brain chemicals dopamine and norepinephrine. Bupropion is available only by prescription.

Following these steps can help you quit using tobacco for good:

Step 1: Do your homework. That way you'll know what to expect. You may experience physical withdrawal symptoms for at least 10 days. Common symptoms include irritability, anxiety and loss of concentration. Afterward, you may still have the urge to light up in familiar smoking situations, such as after a meal or while driving. These urges are generally very brief, but they can be very strong.

By knowing what to expect and having alternative activities planned, you'll be better prepared to handle the urges. These activities might include chewing gum after a meal or snacking on carrot sticks or pretzels when you need to keep your hands busy.

Step 2: Set a stop date. For some people, quitting cold turkey works better than cutting down gradually. Carefully select a date to quit smoking.

Many smokers choose to quit during vacation or while on a trip when they're away from their usual routines and smoking situations. One reason is that your routine changes on vacation. It's easier to break free of smoking rituals when you're away than when you're at work or home.

Step 3: Tell others about your decision. Having the support of family, friends and co-workers can help you reach your goal more quickly. However, many smokers keep their plans to quit a secret because they don't want to look like a failure if they go back to smoking. Many people try three or more times before they're successful, so don't give up.

Step 4: Start changing your routine. Before your stop date, cut down on the number of places you smoke. For instance, stop smoking in your car, and smoke in only one room of the house or outside. This approach will help reduce your smoking urges so that you can be more comfortable in those places without smoking.

Step 5: Talk with your doctor about medications. Nicotine is a highly addictive substance. Withdrawal from nicotine can cause irritability, anxiety and difficulty concentrating. Medications are available that can help lessen withdrawal symptoms and increase your chances of being successful.

Step 6: Take one day at a time. On your stop day, quit completely. Each day, focus your attention on remaining tobacco-free.

Step 7: Avoid smoking situations. Leave the table immediately after meals if this is the time you used to light up. Take a walk instead. If you smoked while using the telephone, avoid long phone conversations or change the place where you talk. If you had a favorite smoking chair, avoid it.

You'll soon be able to anticipate when the urge to smoke will hit you. Before it hits, start doing something that makes smoking inconvenient, such as washing your car or doing relaxation exercises. Your smoking behavior is deeply ingrained and automatic. You need to anticipate your reflex behavior and plan alternatives.

Step 8: Time each urge. Check your watch when a smoking urge hits. Most are short. Once you realize this, it's easier to resist. Tell yourself, "I can make it another few minutes and then the urge will pass."

Expressing your sexuality

Sexuality is a natural and healthy part of living, and a part of your identity as a man or woman. It involves the timeless desire for both physical and emotional intimacy.

Sexuality can be expressed through shared interests, companionship or holding hands. A more physical expression of sexuality is physical contact, including sexual intercourse.

When chronic pain invades your life, the pleasures of sexuality often disappear. You may not feel like socializing, sharing your thoughts and feelings or having close contact. Perhaps you feel your pain has made you less desirable to your partner. Your sleeping arrangement may even have changed. Some people sleep in a spare bedroom or a lounger because they have difficulty getting comfortable or they don't want to keep their partner awake.

In spite of your pain, you can have a healthy and satisfying sexual relationship. It begins with honest communication. You and your partner need to talk about how you feel, what you miss and what you want or need from your relationship. You also need to be creative and willing to make changes. That could be as basic as purchasing a new mattress or a bigger bed so that you don't have to sleep apart, or exploring different ways to express your sexuality.

Making love creatively

Sexual intercourse is just one way to satisfy your need for human closeness. Intimacy can be expressed in many different ways.

Touch. Exploring your partner's body through touch is an exciting way to express your sexual feelings. This can include cuddling, fondling, stroking, massaging and kissing. Touch in any form increases feelings of intimacy.

Self-stimulation. Masturbation is a normal and healthy way to fulfill your sexual needs. One partner may use masturbation during mutual sexual activity if the other partner is unable to be very active.

Oral sex. It can be an alternative or supplement to traditional intercourse.

Timing. A change in the time of day you have sexual intercourse may improve your lovemaking. Many people often have higher pain levels in the evening. If this is true for you, you and your partner might try intercourse in the morning or afternoon.

Experiment with different positions. Lie side by side, kneel or sit. There are many good books available in bookstores that describe different ways to have intercourse.

Vibrators and lubricants. A vibrator can add pleasure without physical exertion. If lack of natural lubrication is a problem, over-the-counter lubricants can prevent pain associated with vaginal dryness.

In all partnerships it takes effort to maintain what is good and to correct what isn't. A healthy sexual relationship can positively affect all aspects of your life, including your physical health, self-esteem, productivity and other relationships.

Becoming more intimate

Start slowly. Before concentrating on improving your sexual relationship, spend time talking. Get to know one another again. Also look for ways to rekindle your romance. Go on a date, plan a picnic, send flowers or exchange personal gifts.

Remind yourself that problems are also opportunities. In your efforts to become more intimate you may discover something about your partner you otherwise might have missed. The relationship you recover may be even better than the one you had before your pain.

Fears about resuming sexual intercourse

You or your partner may have unspoken fears regarding sexual contact and, because of this, may avoid intimate encounters. Delaying intimacy only increases the anxiety surrounding sexual intercourse. Talking openly with your partner about your fears can help ease them.

Fear of increased pain. It's natural to want to avoid additional pain. And it's common to worry that sexual intercourse will cause you physical pain, especially if your pain is centered in your back, abdomen or pelvis.

Experimenting with different positions and other ways to satisfy your and your partner's sexual needs can help the two of you enjoy intimate encounters (see "Making love creatively" on previous page). Relaxation exercises before and after intercourse may help reduce fears and manage pain.

Fear of partner rejection. This is a common feeling. You may wonder if your partner is less attracted to you because of your pain. The longer you have these fears, the more difficult it may be to overcome them. Talk openly with your partner about your feelings and fears and encourage your partner to do the same.

Fear of failure to perform. If you're having difficulty becoming sexually aroused, maintaining an erection or achieving an orgasm, talk with your doctor. Your pain itself, depression, concern over your physical appearance, alcohol and medications all can affect your sexual performance. Many medications, including antidepressants, sedatives and opioids can reduce your sexual ability, including making you impotent. If you suspect a medication may be affecting your sexual performance, don't stop taking the drug without first consulting your doctor.

Sometimes, failure to perform is simply a result of stress and anxiety. Patience and understanding can often help you overcome the problem.

Addressing your spiritual needs

The role of spirituality is an important aspect of well-being that's sometimes overlooked. It may be confused with organized religion, but spirituality is as much connected with the spirit and the soul as it is with any specific belief or form of worship. Spirituality is about meaning, values and purpose in life.

Religion may be one way of expressing spirituality, but it's not the only way. For some people, spirituality is feeling in tune with nature and the universe. For still others, spirituality is expressed through music, meditation or art.

Addressing your spiritual needs can be an effective strategy for managing chronic pain. People find it brings inner peace and added strength to deal with their pain and stress.

Spirituality and healing

Numerous studies have attempted to measure the effect of spirituality on illness and recovery. In reviewing many of these studies, researchers at Georgetown University School of Medicine found that at least 80 percent of the studies suggested spiritual beliefs have a beneficial effect on health. The researchers concluded that people who consider themselves to be spiritual live longer, recover from illness more quickly and with fewer complications, suffer less depression and chemical addiction, have lower blood pressure and cope better with serious disease, such as cancer and cardiovascular disease.

No one knows exactly how spirituality affects health. Some experts attribute the healing effect to hope, which is known to benefit your immune system. Others liken spiritual acts and beliefs to meditation, and still others point to the social connectedness spirituality often provides.

It's important to remember that although spirituality is associated with healing, it isn't a cure. Spirituality can help you live life more fully despite your symptoms, but studies haven't found that it actually cures health problems. It's best to view spirituality as a helpful force, but not a substitute for traditional medical care.

Chapter 16

Staying in control

Throughout this book you've read about ways to help reduce your pain and improve your quality of life. Perhaps you've already begun incorporating these changes into your daily routine. But do you worry about maintaining the progress you're making? What happens when you're confronted with a difficult day?

No doubt, you'll have difficult days. And there may be times when you catch yourself reverting to old habits. You can lessen the effects of these occasional setbacks by developing strategies that help keep you focused on your pain management goals.

10 ways to maintain your gains

To stay in control of your pain, regularly use the pain management strategies outlined in this book, such as exercise, moderation and relaxation. The more you use them, the more beneficial they'll become.

To maintain your progress and avoid relapses:

1. Follow through on your goals
Select your areas of greatest concern, then set some specific, measurable and realistic goals to help you deal with those issues. You

might be worried, for example, that you'll slip back into your old pain behaviors, such as moaning, complaining or limping. Or maybe you're concerned about keeping up your exercise program.

Create a list and check off each goal you reach. To strengthen your motivation, ask a family member or a friend to periodically review your checklist.

2. Monitor your progress
Tracking your accomplishments can motivate you to continue to your goals. Use charts or some other way to display your progress.

3. Make a contract with yourself
Some people find that making a personal commitment to improving their lives and managing their pain helps them follow through with their plans. More than just a goal, a contract becomes a pledge associated with other binding agreements you've made throughout your life.

4. Plan your day
When you specifically schedule time for something — such as exercise or going to a movie — you're more likely to do it. Also use to-do lists or notes on a calendar to remind you of your priorities.

5. Keep your surroundings positive
Look around your house and get rid of things that might lure you back into unhealthy habits. For example, is your bed still sitting in the living room to avoid having to walk upstairs to your bedroom? Are the drapes pulled to keep your rooms dark? Make your house feel like a home, not a hospital. When you walk around your house, you want to see evidence of a person who lives a happy and active life.

6. Seek and accept support
Accepting help from others isn't a sign of weakness, nor does it mean that you're failing. You need support from others to keep you on track and to help you when you have difficult days. In addition

to asking for support from family and friends, consider joining a chronic pain support group.

7. Work with your doctor

Your doctor can be one of your biggest advocates. Keep your doctor updated on your progress and any obstacles you may encounter. He or she can often help you overcome those obstacles.

8. Stay positive

List as many positive statements about yourself as you can and say them to yourself when you're feeling discouraged or in danger of slipping back into some of your old patterns of unhealthy behavior. If you do have a relapse, accept that it happens and move on again, positively.

9. Prepare for challenging situations

Make a list of situations that could disrupt the positive changes you've made. Prepare a response plan that you can use when needed.

Perhaps you've been walking for 30 minutes each day, but you know the weather will soon be changing and you don't like being outside in the snow or cold. How do you still fit in your walk? One option might be to walk indoors at a nearby mall. Or perhaps a local school allows indoor walking during certain hours. You might also consider buying a treadmill.

Another example might be a change at work. You know that your job is going to change and that you'll be taking on new responsibilities. That worries you. One way you might make the transition easier is by developing a list ahead of time. Write down all of the new things you'll need to learn. Prioritize the list and decide what steps you need to take to learn each task. Knowing ahead of time exactly what you need to do and how you're going to do it can make the transition less stressful.

10. Reward yourself

Rewards are a great way to reinforce positive change. When you reach a goal or successfully execute one of your pain strategies, treat yourself to something enjoyable.

Getting through a difficult day

Everyone has a bad day now and then. Holidays can be difficult. Then there's bill time, or an unpredicted, overnight 10-inch snowfall. A visit from relatives also may qualify.

Whatever the reason for your bad day, you can get through it. One of the best ways to minimize the disruptiveness of a tough day and quickly get back to your usual activities is to plan for it. The time to plan for a difficult day is when you're having a good day. On a bad day, it's often difficult to think of ways to cope with the problem. In fact, it can be challenging to concentrate on much of anything except the reason behind the day's souring effect.

Here's how to plan ahead for a difficult day:

Identify sources of your difficult days. Knowing the most common reasons for your difficult days will help you better prepare for them. Think about some recent bad days. Was there a reason for your increased pain? Could it be from too much stress, overdoing it on the weekends, traveling or lack of exercise?

Identify your warning signs. Do you get a warning sign that a bad day is beginning, such as a headache, excessive fatigue or onset of the blues?

Develop a game plan. When you know a difficult day is coming or you get a warning sign, you can lessen its effects by structuring that day with activities and diversions. Having a written plan can help. Your game plan may include some of the following strategies:

Maintain a normal schedule. A difficult day is not a time to overdo it — or to do nothing. Lying around won't help your pain improve or the day go by any faster.

Get out of the house. When you're hurting, it's natural to want to be alone and tend your wounds. But this only gives you more opportunity to think about your pain. Go shopping or visit a friend who can keep you occupied. But steer your conversations away from your pain.

Seek other diversions. Read something enjoyable. Watch a funny movie or call a friend who has a good sense of humor.

Try to relax. On a difficult day, spend more time practicing relaxation techniques, such as listening to tapes or practicing breathing.

Keep away from medication. If you've weaned yourself from medication, don't let a bad day tempt you into taking it again. Remind yourself that it's only a temporary solution and that you're better off without it. If you're taking medication, don't change the dose in an attempt to reduce the pain. You only increase your risk of side effects, and the increased dose may not help your pain.

Say, "This will pass." Because it will.

Joining a support group

Support groups can provide a depth of help and advice and a sense of control that you might not find anywhere else. That's because they put you face to face with people who share many of the same symptoms and feelings that you do.

Not all support groups are the same. Some support groups are mostly educational and feature discussions led by informed guest speakers. Others are more social and unstructured, with meetings providing a time to vent, encourage and visit.

What support groups offer

Benefits of support groups include:

A sense of belonging, of fitting in. There's a special bond between people whose lives have been disrupted by the same problem. You share a sense of camaraderie. Once you experience how others accept you just as you are, you begin to feel more accepting of yourself.

People who understand what you're going through. Family, friends and doctors can sympathize with your problems, but they often can't empathize because they haven't experienced what you have. Your pain experience is unique, but it has many common threads. Support group members have a good idea of what you're feeling and experiencing. Because of this, you feel freer to talk about your frustrations, disappointments and anger.

Exchange of advice. You may be skeptical of the advice friends give you because they don't have chronic pain. But when veteran group members talk, you know they speak with first-hand experience. They can tell you about coping techniques that work for them.

Opportunity to make new friends. These friends can bring joy into your life as well as practical support — a listener when you need to talk or a companion to exercise with.

When support groups aren't the answer

Support groups aren't for everyone. To gain the most benefit from a group, you have to be willing to share your thoughts and feelings. You must also be willing to learn about and help others. People who are severely depressed and don't want to talk or who have poor social skills are generally less likely to benefit from support groups.

In addition, not all support groups are beneficial. You want to be in a group where the mood is upbeat and the message is positive. Some group meetings that aren't carefully monitored can become settings in which to vent and share only negative feelings that feed on themselves.

How to find a support group

Your community may already have one or more support groups for people with chronic pain. There may even be groups for specific types of chronic pain, such as arthritis, fibromyalgia or irritable bowel syndrome.

To find out if there's a support group in your community, check with your doctor or nurse. You might also check with your county health department, a community health organization or your local library. You can also contact organizations such as the American Chronic Pain Association or the National Chronic Pain Outreach Association. (See "Additional resources" on page 191.) These agencies offer free information on area support groups. They can also provide information and advice on how to start a support group if there isn't one in your community.

Support groups and the many other strategies and techniques outlined in this book are designed to help you better understand how pain works and how to live more independently while managing your pain. The more active and productive you can become, the happier you'll be and the better you'll feel.

Your personal planner

Planning your day can help you find a healthier balance for your daily routine. Use this daily planner to schedule your day from the time you wake up until you go to bed. You can plan a day at a time or make your plans for several days.

Each day, include a mix of work, rest, exercise, relaxation and social activity. If you have trouble fitting everything in, ask yourself these three questions:

What do I have to do today? That might include going to work, making it to a scheduled appointment or getting some exercise.

What would be best done today? These are things you don't have to do, but will need your attention at some point. This might include doing a load of laundry, catching up on your bookwork or completing a project at work. Instead of having these activities pile up, it's best to try to spread them out over the week.

What do I want to do today? It's important to spend a certain amount of time each day doing things you enjoy and that help you relax. This could be working in your flower bed, playing a round of golf, visiting with a friend or reading a good book.

Include at least one response to each of these questions as you plan your day. If you're unsure of your plans on certain days, mark as best you can what you think you may be doing. To help you stay on track, refer to your planner throughout the day. Periodically write down what you did and compare it with your plan.

If you find that scheduling your day helps you to achieve your goals, then continue to do so. You can purchase a daily planner at most office supply stores and many bookstores. Or, you can make your own. However, once you get into a routine, you may find that you don't need to be as detailed in your planning. Marking down a few key times or events may be all that you need to do.

On the following page is a sample day to give you an idea of the information you might include in your daily schedule.

Day: *Thursday*

Date: *May 10*

	I plan to	**I did**
6:00 a.m.	*Exercise, eat breakfast*	*Exercised, ate breakfast*
7:00 a.m.	*Clean up and leave for work*	*Got ready and went to work*
8:00 a.m.	*Finish letters from yesterday*	*Letters*
9:00 a.m.	*Complete letters*	*Letters, worked on meeting agenda*
10:00 a.m.	*Start work on new files*	*Letters*
11:00 a.m.	*New files*	*Started new files*
12:00 p.m.	*Meet Susan for lunch*	*Lunch with Susan*
1:00 p.m.	*Continue work on files*	*New files*
2:00 p.m.	*Department meeting*	*Meeting*
3:00 p.m.	*Complete files*	*Meeting follow-up*
4:00 p.m.	*Make phone calls, other details*	*Phone calls, memos, etc.*
5:00 p.m.	*Go home, rest, ride bike*	*Went home, rested, rode bike*
6:00 p.m.	*Prepare and eat dinner*	*Dinner*
7:00 p.m.	*Do laundry and iron*	*Laundry, rested*
8:00 p.m.	*Work on class reunion schedule*	*Ironed, visited with Louise*
9:00 p.m.	*Relaxation exercises, rest*	*Relaxation exercises, helped Jeff*
10:00 p.m.	*Read book, go to bed*	*Read book and went to bed*
11:00 p.m.	*Sleep*	*Slept*

Day: _____

Date: _____

	I plan to	I did
6:00 a.m.		
7:00 a.m.		
8:00 a.m.		
9:00 a.m.		
10:00 a.m.		
11:00 a.m.		
12:00 p.m.		
1:00 p.m.		
2:00 p.m.		
3:00 p.m.		
4:00 p.m.		
5:00 p.m.		
6:00 p.m.		
7:00 p.m.		
8:00 p.m.		
9:00 p.m.		
10:00 p.m.		
11:00 p.m.		

PERSONAL **PLANNER**

Day: _____

Date: _____

	I plan to	I did
6:00 a.m.		
7:00 a.m.		
8:00 a.m.		
9:00 a.m.		
10:00 a.m.		
11:00 a.m.		
12:00 p.m.		
1:00 p.m.		
2:00 p.m.		
3:00 p.m.		
4:00 p.m.		
5:00 p.m.		
6:00 p.m.		
7:00 p.m.		
8:00 p.m.		
9:00 p.m.		
10:00 p.m.		
11:00 p.m.		

PERSONAL PLANNER

Day: _____

Date: _____

	I plan to	I did
6:00 a.m.		
7:00 a.m.		
8:00 a.m.		
9:00 a.m.		
10:00 a.m.		
11:00 a.m.		
12:00 p.m.		
1:00 p.m.		
2:00 p.m.		
3:00 p.m.		
4:00 p.m.		
5:00 p.m.		
6:00 p.m.		
7:00 p.m.		
8:00 p.m.		
9:00 p.m.		
10:00 p.m.		
11:00 p.m.		

PERSONAL **PLANNER**

Day: _____

Date: _____

	I plan to	**I did**
6:00 a.m.		
7:00 a.m.		
8:00 a.m.		
9:00 a.m.		
10:00 a.m.		
11:00 a.m.		
12:00 p.m.		
1:00 p.m.		
2:00 p.m.		
3:00 p.m.		
4:00 p.m.		
5:00 p.m.		
6:00 p.m.		
7:00 p.m.		
8:00 p.m.		
9:00 p.m.		
10:00 p.m.		
11:00 p.m.		

Day: _____

Date: _____

	I plan to	**I did**
6:00 a.m.		
7:00 a.m.		
8:00 a.m.		
9:00 a.m.		
10:00 a.m.		
11:00 a.m.		
12:00 p.m.		
1:00 p.m.		
2:00 p.m.		
3:00 p.m.		
4:00 p.m.		
5:00 p.m.		
6:00 p.m.		
7:00 p.m.		
8:00 p.m.		
9:00 p.m.		
10:00 p.m.		
11:00 p.m.		

PERSONAL PLANNER

Day: _____

Date: _____

	I plan to	**I did**
6:00 a.m.		
7:00 a.m.		
8:00 a.m.		
9:00 a.m.		
10:00 a.m.		
11:00 a.m.		
12:00 p.m.		
1:00 p.m.		
2:00 p.m.		
3:00 p.m.		
4:00 p.m.		
5:00 p.m.		
6:00 p.m.		
7:00 p.m.		
8:00 p.m.		
9:00 p.m.		
10:00 p.m.		
11:00 p.m.		

PERSONAL PLANNER

Day: _____

Date: _____

	I plan to	**I did**
6:00 a.m.	_____	_____
7:00 a.m.	_____	_____
8:00 a.m.	_____	_____
9:00 a.m.	_____	_____
10:00 a.m.	_____	_____
11:00 a.m.	_____	_____
12:00 p.m.	_____	_____
1:00 p.m.	_____	_____
2:00 p.m.	_____	_____
3:00 p.m.	_____	_____
4:00 p.m.	_____	_____
5:00 p.m.	_____	_____
6:00 p.m.	_____	_____
7:00 p.m.	_____	_____
8:00 p.m.	_____	_____
9:00 p.m.	_____	_____
10:00 p.m.	_____	_____
11:00 p.m.	_____	_____

PERSONAL **PLANNER**

Day: _____

Date: _____

	I plan to	**I did**
6:00 a.m.	_____	_____
7:00 a.m.	_____	_____
8:00 a.m.	_____	_____
9:00 a.m.	_____	_____
10:00 a.m.	_____	_____
11:00 a.m.	_____	_____
12:00 p.m.	_____	_____
1:00 p.m.	_____	_____
2:00 p.m.	_____	_____
3:00 p.m.	_____	_____
4:00 p.m.	_____	_____
5:00 p.m.	_____	_____
6:00 p.m.	_____	_____
7:00 p.m.	_____	_____
8:00 p.m.	_____	_____
9:00 p.m.	_____	_____
10:00 p.m.	_____	_____
11:00 p.m.	_____	_____

Additional resources

Contact these organizations for more information about chronic pain or associated conditions. Some groups offer free printed materials or videos. Others have publications or videos you can purchase.

American Academy of Craniofacial Pain

520 West Pipeline Road
Hurst, Texas 76053
817-282-1501
www.aacfp.org

American Academy of Orofacial Pain

19 Mantua Road
Mount Royal, NJ 08061
856-423-3629
www.aaop.org

American Academy of Pain Medicine

4700 West Lake Avenue
Glenview, IL 60025
847-375-4731
www.painmed.org

American Chronic Pain Association

P.O. Box 850
Rocklin, CA 95677
916-632-0922
www.theacpa.org

American Council for Headache Education

19 Mantua Road
Mount Royal, NJ 08061
800-255-2243 or 856-423-0258
www.achenet.org

American Fibromyalgia Syndrome Association, Inc.

6380 East Tanque Verde, Suite D
Tucson, AZ 85715
520-733-1570
www.afsafund.org

American Headache Society

19 Mantua Road
Mount Royal, NJ 08061
856-423-0043
www.ahsnet.org

American Pain Foundation

210 North Charles Street
Suite 710
Baltimore, MD 21201-4111
888-615-7246
www.painfoundation.org

American Pain Society

4700 West Lake Avenue
Glenview, IL 60025
847-375-4715
Fax: 877-734-8758
www.ampainsoc.org

Arthritis Foundation

P.O. Box 7669
Atlanta, GA 30357-0669
800-283-7800
www.arthritis.org

Endometriosis Association

8585 North 76th Place
Milwaukee, WI 53223
800-992-3636 or 414-355-2200
www.endometriosisassn.org

Fibromyalgia Network

P.O. Box 31750
Tucson, AZ 85751-1750
800-853-2929
www.fmnetnews.com

International Association for the Study of Pain

909 Northeast 43rd Street
Suite 306
Seattle, WA 98105
206-547-6409
www.iasp-pain.org

International Foundation for Functional Gastrointestinal Disorders

P.O. Box 170864
Milwaukee, WI 53217
888-964-2001 or 414-964-1799
www.iffgd.org

Interstitial Cystitis Association

110 North Washington Street
Suite 340
Rockville, MD 20850
301-610-5300
www.ichelp.org

Mayo Clinic Health Information

www.MayoClinic.com

National Center for Complementary and Alternative Medicine

P.O. Box 7934
Gaithersburg, MD 20898
888-644-6226
nccam.nih.gov

National Chronic Pain Outreach Association

P.O. Box 274
Milboro, VA 24460
540-862-9437

National Headache Foundation
428 West St. James Place, 2nd Floor
Chicago, IL 60614
888-643-5552
www.headaches.org

National Pain Foundation
P.O. Box 102605
Denver, CO 80250
303-756-0889
www.painconnection.org

Neuropathy Association
60 East 42nd Street
Suite 942
New York, NY 10165-0999
800-247-6968 or 212-692-0662
www.neuropathy.org

Reflex Sympathetic Dystrophy Syndrome Association
P.O. Box 502
Milford, CT 06460
203-877-3790
www.rsds.org

TMJ Association, Ltd
P.O. Box 26770
Milwaukee, WI 53226
414-259-3223
www.tmj.org

Trigeminal Neuralgia Association
2801 Southwest Archer Road
Suite C
Gainesville, FL 32608
352-376-9955
www.tna-support.org

Glossary

addiction. An illness in which a person seeks and consumes a substance, such as alcohol, tobacco or a drug, despite the fact that it causes harm.

aerobic (are-O-bik) **exercise.** *Aerobic* means "with oxygen." In reference to exercise, the term refers to the intensity and duration of activity and the energy fuel being used.

allodynia (al-o-DIN-e-uh). An altered sensation in which normally nonpainful events are felt as pain.

analgesic (an-ul-JE-zik). A medication or agent that reduces pain.

anesthetic. A substance used to abolish sensation.

anticonvulsant. A drug used to prevent seizures, which also may be useful for treating pain.

autonomic nervous system. The portion of the nervous system that regulates involuntary body functions, including those of the heart and intestine. Controls blood flow, digestion and temperature regulation.

bursa. A fluid-containing sac near or involving a joint or bony prominence that reduces friction between a tendon and a bone, or between a bone and skin during movement.

celiac plexus (SE-le-ak PLEK-sus). A network of nerve fibers in the abdomen that's controlled by the autonomic nervous system. This group of nerves also conducts pain sensation from the abdominal organs, such as the liver, spleen, stomach and pancreas.

corticosteroids. Anti-inflammatory drugs created from or based on a naturally occurring hormone (cortisone) produced by the cortex of the adrenal glands.

cortisone. A naturally occurring hormone produced by the cortex of the adrenal glands. It decreases inflammation.

COX-2 inhibitor. A nonsteroidal anti-inflammatory drug (NSAID) that specifically inhibits an enzyme known as cyclooxygenase-2 (COX-2). These drugs are used to treat pain and may be less likely to cause gastrointestinal bleeding than other NSAIDs.

dysthesia. An unpleasant, abnormal sensation, often described as burning or crawling. May be spontaneous or evoked.

endorphins. Naturally occurring molecules made up of amino acids. Endorphins attach to special receptors in the brain and spinal cord to stop pain messages. These are the same receptors that respond to morphine.

enkephalins (en-KEF-uh-lins). Naturally occurring molecules in the brain. Enkephalins attach to special receptors in your brain and spinal cord to stop pain messages. They also affect other functions within the brain and nervous system.

epidural anesthesia. A procedure used to provide anesthesia during labor and some surgery. Medication is given through a catheter placed in the back. Also called an epidural block.

ergonomics. The science of designing the job to fit the worker, rather than physically forcing the worker's body to fit the job.

facet joint (FAS-ut joint). A joint between two adjacent vertebrae. Each vertebra is connected at the intervertebral disk in the front and the two facet joints in the back.

field block injection. A procedure used to relax a muscle or to reduce muscle pain and inflammation. The targeted muscle is injected with a local anesthetic and corticosteroid. Also called trigger point injection.

frontal cortex. The portion of the brain that's involved with reasoning, planning, abstract thought and other complex cognitive functions in addition to motor function.

hyperalgesia. Abnormally increased pain sensation.

inflammation. The protective response of body tissues to irritation or injury. Inflammation may be acute or chronic. Signs and symptoms are redness, heat, swelling and pain, often accompanied by loss of function.

intraspinal. Within or into the vertebral column, which contains the spinal cord and cerebrospinal fluid.

limbic system. The portion of the brain that produces emotions.

local anesthetic. A medication that blocks electrical signals in nerves. It eliminates pain in a specific part of the body and causes intended, temporary paralysis.

myofascial pain. Pain and tenderness in the muscles and adjacent fibrous tissues (fascia).

narcotics. A group of drugs that relieves pain by preventing transmission of pain messages to the brain. Also referred to as opioids.

nerve block. A local anesthetic that is injected around a nerve, preventing pain messages traveling along that nerve pathway from reaching the brain. Used most often to relieve pain for a short period, such as during a surgery.

neuralgia. Pain that extends along one or more nerve pathways.

neurobiology. A branch of biology that is concerned with the anatomy and physiology of the nervous system.

neurolytic. A substance or procedure that destroys nerves.

neuromodulation. Electrical stimulation of a peripheral nerve, the spinal cord or the brain for relief of pain. It may be done transcutaneously or with an implanted stimulator.

neuropathic pain. Pain that originates from a damaged nerve or nervous system.

neurotransmitters. Chemicals in the brain, such as acetylcholine, serotonin and norepinephrine, that facilitate communication between nerve cells (neurons).

nociceptors (no-sih-SEP-turs). Nerve endings attached to peripheral nerves that detect potential or actual tissue damage. They sense unpleasant situations such as extreme heat, cold, a cut or pressure.

nonsteroidal anti-inflammatory drugs (NSAIDS). (en-SAYDS). Medications used to reduce inflammation that aren't corticosteroid based.

occupational therapy. Skilled treatment that helps people return to ordinary tasks around home and at work by maximizing physical potential through lifestyle adaptations and possible use of assistive devices.

pain behaviors. Responses to pain that include talking about pain, rubbing or protecting an affected part of the body, or avoiding routine activities because of pain.

pain scale. A system of rating pain. Often based on a scale of 0 to 10, with 0 being no pain and 10 being the worst pain imaginable.

pain threshold. The point at which pain is noticeable.

pain tolerance level. The peak amount of pain that a person can endure.

palliative care. Care given to people with chronic, often life-threatening illnesses. Care focuses on symptom management, such as relieving pain or stopping nausea, enhancing quality of life and psychosocial needs.

patient controlled analgesia (PCA). A system that allows people to control the amount of pain medication that they receive. The person pushes a button and a machine delivers a dose of pain medicine into the bloodstream through a vein.

peripheral nerves. Nerves that run from your spinal cord to all other parts of your body. Peripheral nerves transmit messages from the spinal cord and the brain to and from other parts of your body, and send sensory signals back to the spinal cord and brain.

phantom pain. Pain or discomfort following amputation that feels as if it comes from the missing limb.

physiatrist. A doctor who specializes in physical medicine and rehabilitation. A physiatrist evaluates and recommends treatments that restore function in people with chronic disease.

physical dependence. The physical condition in which rapid discontinuation of a substance, such as alcohol, tobacco or a drug, causes a withdrawal reaction.

physical therapist. A trained professional who teaches exercises and other physical activities to aid in rehabilitation and maximize physical ability with less pain.

rebound pain. When regular use of a pain medication makes a person's pain worse instead of better.

receptors. Located on the outer side of a receiving nerve cell, receptors bind the neurotransmitter to the receiving nerve cell and change the activity of this cell.

reflex sympathetic dystrophy (RSD). A chronic and painful condition that usually affects an arm or leg. Signs and symptoms include intense burning or aching pain along with swelling, abnormal sweating and hypersensitivity of the area.

regional anesthesia. Medications used to block pain in a certain region of the body without altering consciousness.

sciatica. Achiness that may include tingling, numbness or muscle weakness along the sciatic nerve. This major nerve runs through the buttock muscles into the back of the thigh and divides into two nerves behind the knee that run down into the foot.

selective serotonin reuptake inhibitors (SSRIs). Medications used to relieve depression. May work by increasing the availability of a brain chemical that helps to regulate mood (serotonin).

serotonin (ser-o-TOE-nin). A brain chemical (neurotransmitter) that helps to regulate your mood. A lack of it may lead to depression.

somatosensory cortex. A part of the brain responsible for processing stimulation coming from the skin, body wall, muscles, bones, tendons and joints. It plays a part in determining pain intensity.

spinal nerve block. A procedure that's used to relieve pain affecting a broad area, such as the abdomen or the legs. A local anesthetic is injected in or near the spinal column, preventing pain messages traveling along that nerve pathway from reaching the brain.

stellate ganglion block. A procedure designed to relieve pain caused by overactivity of the sympathetic nervous system in the upper extremities, the head or the neck. A local anesthetic is injected into the front of the neck to block sympathetic nerves without blocking sensory pathways.

substance P. A protein substance that stimulates nerve endings at an injury site and within the spinal cord, increasing pain messages.

sympathetic block. An injection of an anesthetic to relieve pain resulting from abnormal activity of the sympathetic nervous system. The sympathetic nerves control circulation and perspiration and are part of your autonomic nervous system.

syndrome. A collection of symptoms that characterize a specific disease or condition.

thalamus. A portion of the brain that relays impulses from the sensory nerves. Sensory nerves enable people to feel objects that they touch, and they allow people to feel pain.

tolerance. The point at which a person adapts to a specific substance, so larger amounts of the prescribed medication or a new medication is needed to achieve the same results.

topical agents. Medications that are applied to the skin rather than ingested or injected. They can come in the form of a cream or a gel. Also called ointments.

transdermal. Entering via the skin, such as a medicated cream being absorbed through the skin.

tricyclic antidepressants. A group of drugs used to relieve symptoms of depression. These drugs may also help relieve pain.

trigger point. Places on the body where muscles and adjacent fibrous tissue (fascia) are sensitive to touch. These areas are generally in the upper and lower back muscles, but they may occur elsewhere.

withdrawal. The physical or psychological state experienced when certain substances or medications are discontinued rapidly.

Index

Note: Glossary definitions are indicated by the **boldface** page numbers.

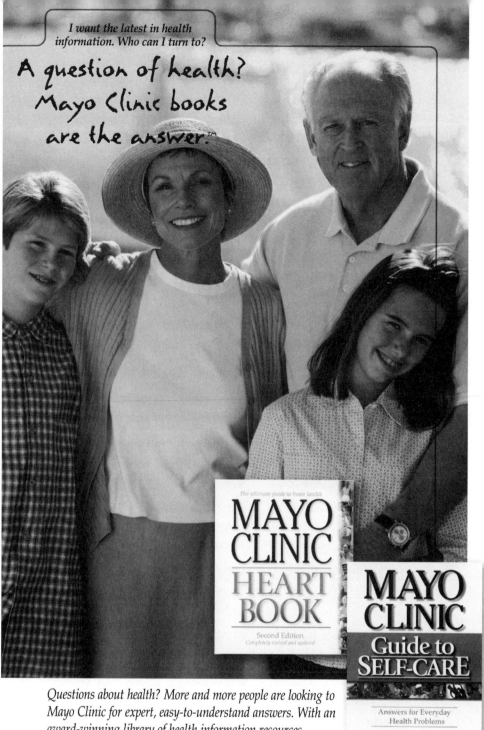

I want the latest in health information. Who can I turn to?

A question of health? Mayo Clinic books are the answer.

The ultimate guide to heart health

MAYO CLINIC HEART BOOK

Second Edition
Completely revised and updated

MAYO CLINIC Guide to SELF-CARE

Answers for Everyday Health Problems

Questions about health? More and more people are looking to Mayo Clinic for expert, easy-to-understand answers. With an award-winning library of health information resources — including a Web site, books and newsletters — reliable answers to your health questions can be right at your fingertips.

www.MayoClinic.com

© 2002, Mayo Foundation for Medical Education and Research.

When you purchase Mayo Clinic newsletters and books, proceeds are used to further medical education and research at Mayo Clinic. You not only get answers to your questions on health, but become part of the solution.

Arthritis doesn't have to rule your life!

Arthritis can be disabling, but it doesn't have to defeat you. You can take control of your arthritis with the new information in *Mayo Clinic on Arthritis, Second Edition.*

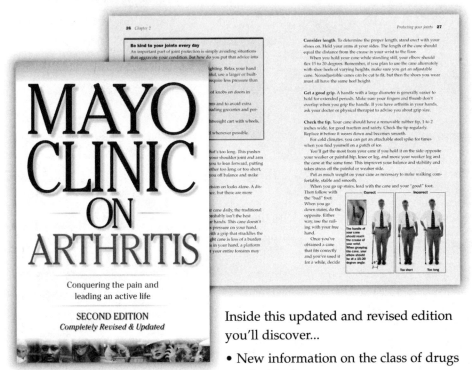

Inside this updated and revised edition you'll discover...

- New information on the class of drugs called biologics.

- New information from Mayo Clinic specialists about complementary and alternative medicine treatments of arthritis.

- New information on surgery, including an update on the effectiveness of hip replacement surgery.

- Where to find reliable arthritis information online.

- Exercises to help you stay fit and flexible.

- How diet can make a difference.

This new second edition contains the best information we know to help you control your arthritis so it doesn't control you!

Mayo Clinic on Arthritis, Second Edition
product # 268502 • **$16.95**

Available at your favorite bookstore, or you may order direct by calling 1-877-647-6397. Order code 251.
(Price does not include shipping, handling or applicable sales tax.)

Mayo Clinic Health Information-providing answers to your questions regarding health.

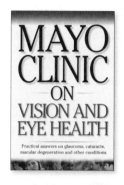

Is your eyesight as good as it could be?

Now learn the latest options from Mayo Clinic on preserving your precious vision and protecting the health of your eyes. *Mayo Clinic on Vision and Eye Health* offers scores of tips and ideas that you and your eye care professional can use to enhance your eye health.

Mayo Clinic on Vision and Eye Health
product #270600 • **$14.95**

Knowledge is the key to dealing with Alzheimer's Disease.

In the last few decades, researchers have made tremendous advances in our understanding of Alzheimer's disease. Physicians are now able to diagnose Alzheimer's at earlier stages and treat symptoms that had previously complicated or hastened mental decline. Learn what the experts at Mayo Clinic tell their patients.

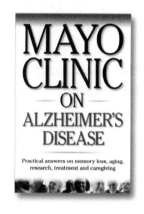

Also included is the QUICK GUIDE FOR CARE-GIVERS, a special reference section providing practical advice for caregivers.

Mayo Clinic on Alzheimer's Disease
product # 270700 • **$16.95**

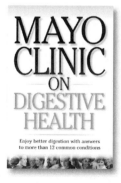

Improve your digestive health!

This book from Mayo Clinic includes more than 190 pages of easy-to-understand information regarding common digestive conditions. You'll learn how to identify, manage and prevent digestive disorders, so you can enjoy life with less stomach and intestinal upset.

Mayo Clinic on Digestive Health
product # 268900 • **$14.95**

Available at your favorite bookstore, or you may order direct by calling 1-877-647-6397. Order code 251.

(Price does not include shipping, handling or applicable sales tax.)

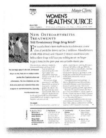
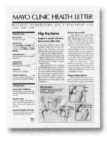
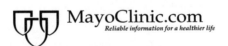